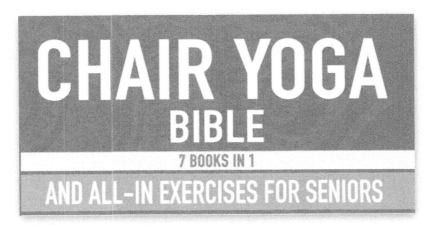

CHAIR YOGA
BIBLE
7 BOOKS IN 1
AND ALL-IN EXERCISES FOR SENIORS

Chair Yoga Poses Workouts, Stretching, Core, Water Aerobics Routines to Strengthen Balance, Recover Well-Being and Falling Prevention

CLAUDINE WELLS

Project manager: WISEGUYSBOOKS

Illustrator: S. Kalpage

ISBN: 9798353765844

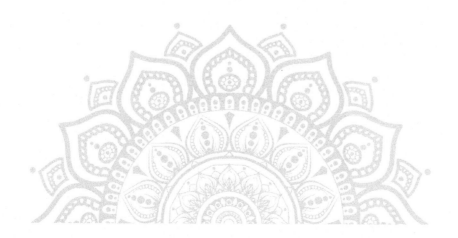

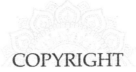

COPYRIGHT

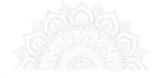

ABOUT THE AUTHOR

Claudine Wells is a 63 years old soul who lives as a Pilates and Yoga instructor for seniors and herbal healer 'nana.'

She has been a senior Yoga teacher for ten years in Bali, where she lives with her husband Mike and Cassandra, her cat that everyone calls 'Cassie', and her beloved turtle Lulù.

Claudine has two kids and one grandchild, who hopefully will soon discover the magic world of Yoga, balance, and spiritual awakening.

She loves writing, gardening, healing with herbs, Yoga retreats, taking and giving lessons, performing Moon's rituals, and going for long walks in Nature.

With an Italian heritage descending from her grandmother, Claudine comes from Minnesota, where she celebrated the snow as a source of inspiration, while she now prefers Indonesian vibes that resonate more with her true spirit.

Before starting reading, Claudine thought of giving you a gift to amplify the experience of the book: a training journal to follow your workouts with awareness and fun!

Download it here using the QR code (in the image below) ...
and stay in touch with Claudine!

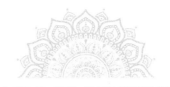

TABLE OF CONTENTS

Book IV: Balance Exercises For Seniors For Falling Prevention

Book V: Water Aerobics and Low Impact Swimming Pool Exercises For Senior

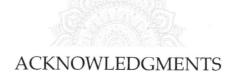

ACKNOWLEDGMENTS

As I reread the draft of this book, my list of people to thank just got longer and longer :)
First, I would like to thank my husband, Mike, for always being my rock, my portal. Over the years, he gave me a loving and protective environment that allowed me to express myself in all respects, even when I informed him of my intention to move to Bali while shoveling 1 meter of snow at our home in Minnesota!
Then, of course, I thank Cassandra, my wonderful and impatient cat. For the occasion of the writing of this book, she has been waiting for her well-deserved cuddles without complaining, scratching the sofa, or bothering my sweet turtle Lulù.
I clearly thank my children, grandchildren, and entire family for having accompanied me over the years with their inner wisdom: each of them has contributed to making me the person - and the Yoga teacher - that I am now.
Thanks to my students from Bali Yoga classes and someone online too! I am happy that the audience of aspiring Yogis is also expanding to the 'less senior' students!
Finally, I thank all those who helped me realize this collection of books: it was a difficult job, but someone had to do it! Thanks to my beloved Wise Guys Crew for the continued research, comfort, and support! And also for inspiring the illustrations in this book, posing for the illustrator and me without complaining! As a giveaway, I took a few years from some of them :)
And last but not least, I thank you: arriving in your home and supporting you on your journey towards well-being and love for yourself is priceless for me! My heart is full of gratitude!

Namasté, Claudine

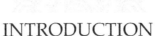

INTRODUCTION

I have been thinking a lot about it: how to start this book collection? I walked the length and breadth of the streets of Pecatu (which in my grandmother's native language sounds like 'sin,' almost as if I wanted to remember my Italian genealogy every day), looking for inspiration.

So much so that my partner literally forced me to sit in the chair and start. So, here I am!

I thought about it a lot, as I said, because I feel honored to be able to accompany you from this moment on, on your journey of discovery of yourself, of your body, of your mind. And also of your spirit.

Yes, why undertake a discipline such as Yoga (even if it is in the version with the chair - do not think even for a moment that it is a sort of 'little sister,' because it is not, and we will see it), or work daily to perform a stretching exercise, or even training your balance to avoid hurting yourself, is not just about the body.

If there's one thing I have understood in all my years of working with senior people - and then I became senior with them too! - it is this: any type of training pushes you beyond the knowledge you have of yourself. Or you think you have, said even more precisely.

Your body, on the other hand, is a perfectly imperfect machine. It works like a foolproof system most of the time, but, like any rule-proving exception, it 'jams' every now and then.

As a mental imprint and a society that is always on the run and connected, we are used to thinking of these moments as a 'bug,' a flaw in a perfect system that needs to be 'fixed.' Then we resort to any system of care and repair that guarantees us a 'button' able to reset that state of perfection in a short time, in an economical and effortless way.

Yet, sadly and fortunately, things don't work out that way. And definitely, our bodies don't work that way.

So I started to see that moment of pure 'imperfection' as a 'sign,' not necessarily negative: our body, which communicates through its intuition, is sending us a message at that exact moment.

And it could be a message that tells us that we are not noticing it, that we are not treating it with respect, or that we are going too fast and must stop and recharge. Whatever this message is, we see it in the form of aches, creaking joints, accidents, falls, or illnesses.

And in this perfectly imperfect communication system, then, how can we respond to the demands of our body: by taking care of it! It is undoubtedly more accessible than all the work the body has to do to send us an SOS signal. All we have to do is begin to know it, touch it, move it and understand it. We must, in practice, learn from it. And the only way we can manage to do that is to connect with it through training.

Our society has given us the wrong idea of training: performing hard and extreme leads to success. Conversely, there is a softer version of moving the body, which becomes ideal when we are 50-60-70 years old (and even more!). It is called gentle or low-impact gymnastics.

And here we are: in this collection of books, you will find the most effective methods to be able to train not only daily with specific and targeted exercises but also to create this state of connection and grace together with your body.

My Italian grandmother always used this expression when she was thrilled, *'non sto più nella pelle,'* which means 'I'm not in my skin anymore.' I love this expression because it almost inspires us to 'transcend' from our physical bodies to touch something that lies beyond. Well: that's precisely what will happen!

With the training, routines, and workouts that you will find inside the book, at the same time, you will be able to work on your training and touch much higher well-being. Your mind, body, and spirit will sail the sea of your senior years with thanks and all together.

Practically speaking, there is so much more at stake than just a senior training program!

By now, the data speak clearly: the average duration of life has increased, and in the coming years, we will see a further increase in this figure. However, it is clear that the goal is not just to live longer but to live longer in health, with energy, and enjoy the benefits that each season of life offers.

To use a well-known expression that represents this concept, 'it is not simply a question of adding more years of life but of adding more life to our years.'

The primary way to achieve this goal is to experience wellness by this expression, adopting a healthy lifestyle and behaviors consisting of proper nutrition, stress management, a positive approach to life, and regular physical activity.

Physical activity is a fundamental pillar of the wellness approach. There is now substantial scientific evidence to support the enormous benefits of physical activity at all ages: from infancy, the age of development, maturity, the third age, and the fourth age.

Physical activity is a protective factor for so-called non-communicable diseases such as cardiovascular disease, stroke, diabetes, obesity and hypertension, and some types of cancer. It also promotes better mental health, delays the onset of dementia, and improves the general quality of life.

All these well-documented benefits are also modulated according to the so-called 'dose-response effect': the higher the frequency and total volume of activity, the greater the advantages in reducing certain diseases and improving health in several critical areas.

However, I don't want to go too far because, in addition to loving philosophical discourses on life and soul, I am also efficient and practical as a true Taurus :) Therefore, let's cut to the chase.

Before describing it in detail, I want to specify that each of the books will first contain a theoretical component to know what you are about to do, the benefits and the excellent help that it is able to give to the elderly, and then a completely practical part with the exercises explained individually and the primary reference workouts.

Here's what you can find in this book collection!

Book 1 - Chair Yoga Exercises For Seniors

The first activity you will find in this collection is Chair Yoga. On the other hand, it could not be otherwise. I consider Yoga (and also Chair Yoga) the 'Queen' of senior training. And this is both from the point of view of the practicality of execution and for the avalanche of health benefits at 360°.

Yoga is the best activity to regain optimal physical balance and, at the same time, clear the mind of any negativity through meditation.

Seniors can approach the practice of Yoga so that they can benefit from the many benefits it offers!

In the book, we will address all the myths and facts that make this discipline a millennial path of well-being at your service. And, obviously, we will discover the best positions on the chair for Beginners and Advanced, as well as the main flows to train us to know Yoga and ourselves a little better every day.

Note: most of the poses in this book are also suitable for wheelchair users. In this regard, you will find a specific flow in Book 7. However, for your convenience, the instructions for learning the positions are in Book 1. Read the instructions carefully, and then... go with the flow... even on your wheelchair!

Chair Yoga: Millennial Paths for Your Happiness.

Book 2 - Stretching Exercises For Seniors

The second type of activity concerns stretching, truly one of the most underestimated moments of training and also one of its main allies.

On the other hand, stretching is genuinely an essential help for the elderly. This type of gymnastics must be practiced in a gentle way, and its main characteristic is to keep the muscles well-oxygenated and the joints flexible thanks to their constant stretching.

Practiced after the training two or three times a week, it preserves the joints and maintains and strengthens the balance, making the life of the elderly more autonomous and safer.

Moreover, practiced correctly and above all constantly, this activity brings tangible benefits in everyday life, making their life qualitatively better.

We will discover together the importance of stretching in the name of flexibility, how to best perform essential exercises, and also the main routines to perform at the right time, even in combination with other workouts.

Stretching: Flexibility is The Key.

Book 3 - Core and Strength Exercises for Seniors

As with stretching, core training also becomes essential during the senior years. On the other hand, in oriental medicine, the core represents our true essence: if it is strong, we are too. This is why for the elderly, having a trained core transforms into power, balance, and strength. Also, representing the connection point between the upper and lower body, the core is responsible for most movements necessary to lead a satisfying life.

Training is, therefore, a priority, which amplifies even more after the age of 50 because it is at that age that the body begins to weaken, requiring a more incisive contrasting action.

In addition to preventing injuries, a more robust midsection helps improve body stability and coordination, counteract back pain, and improve posture and daily movements.

We will train the core with the most important exercises, build many workout routines, and even weekly standing, mat, and sitting patterns.

Core and Strength: Your Inner Power.

Book 4 - Balance Exercises For Seniors For Fall Prevention

One of the main aspects of the health of the elderly is being able to remain firm on their feet. The relationship between seniors and balance is a very delicate relationship. Falls and unstable balance, in fact, are among the most common clinical problems after a certain age and can cause fractures and injuries, which, in a significant percentage of cases, lead to immobilization and are life-threatening.

The more the years pass, the more the chances of falling and, therefore, of getting traumas increase, and this is true for several reasons (we will see them in detail in the book).

Therefore, balance and strength exercises can help prevent falls by improving the ability to control and maintain the position of your body, both during movement and when standing still. No more falls, therefore, and with a few minutes dedicated to the day, this healthy dream can become your next reality.

In addition to the best fall prevention exercises, you will finally find targeted exercises to boost your strength, posture, and flexibility every day and forever.

Balance: Never Falling Again.

Book 5 - Water Aerobics and Low-Impact Pool Exercises For Seniors

Among the elements that make up Mother Earth, water is perhaps the one that 'completes' us most closely. We are concretely made of water; in the water, we are light, pure ethereal.

Furthermore, water is the fundamental element for human health, the leading food we should never neglect for the organism's well-being. That's why training in the water has become a moment of pure well-being, especially for seniors.

The main objective of water training in senior and elderly subjects is to prevent the risk of falling through an improvement in the static and dynamic balance.

In fact, in water, the body's weight decreases drastically, reducing by 90% when the water reaches the level of the neck. In this way, there is less joint discharge, which is beneficial in those subjects with numerous limitations of dry movement and who, on the other hand, can move more freely in the water thanks to the facilitating conditions of this environment.

Finally, a further beneficial effect not to be overlooked is the best psychological approach of the elderly person towards these activities, as demonstrated by these and many other pieces of scientific evidence. In the water, there is no risk of falling and, therefore, the risk of causing any debilitating fractures, which are, as we know, among the significant causes of hospitalization and death in the elderly population.

In the book, we will discover how to train in the water in total safety and relaxation, the best exercises to do, and the routines to train whenever you want.

Water Aerobics: Light and Alive.

Book 6 - All-In Minute Workouts and Exercises For Seniors

Constant and daily training contributes to the development of heart performance with less fatigue and better general self-esteem.

Furthermore, the elderly who train notice from the first weeks an improvement in strength, muscular endurance, and motor coordination, a strengthening of the bones, and an improvement in physical and psychological balance, which allows them to remedy the accelerated rhythm and stress of modern life.

And to do all this, you don't necessarily need long and alienating training. It only takes a few minutes a day, constant and focused, to see tremendous results.

Whether you have 5 minutes, 20 minutes, or an hour, in this book, you can choose the right minute workout for you, depending on your precious time and goal!

Minutes Exercises: Your Time, Your Rules.

Book 7 - W4W: Workouts For Well-Being

Finally, I specifically made the last book that closes our collection for you and for your practicality: all the routines and workouts dedicated to every single problem or physical discomfort you will encounter during your senior years. Programs for pain in general, both at home and in the water, but also specifically dedicated to wheelchair users, those with back pain, arthritis, or fragile knees, those who want to lose some weight, and much more. With the hope, of course, that you never have to browse it!

Well-Being Special Flows: Eternal Joy.

Claudine's Tips

I have conceptualized this book as a 'Bible,' and this word is not here by chance. I have always loved reading books or keeping those texts on the nightstand that, instinctively and holistically, could represent 'everything' or answer any doubts I might have on a particular topic. That's why I chose the word 'Bible' so that you can make this book your own, read it, and love it so that it answers every question regarding training and balance of body, mind, and soul, without having to look for them in hundreds of books in bookstores or online.

Finally, an aspect not to be overlooked is detailed illustrations for each exercise and instructions to perform it in total safety. Of course, it would be very presumptuous to think that EVERYTHING could be in here. However, in an age where information is jagged, and so is our confidence and mental clarity, this book can indeed contain everything you need in order to live your senior years in a happy, smiling, and loving way.

And who knows: maybe you will find yourself having to lend it to your grandchildren or, even better, doing the exercises with them!

So, let's begin!

BOOK 1:
CHAIR YOGA EXERCISES FOR SENIORS

Chapter 1
Millennial Paths for Your Happiness

2022. Yoga has officially entered our daily routine.

This shocking and enlightening millenary practice, after years of knowledge only among insiders, meditation experts, mindfulness enthusiasts, and travellers in search of themselves among the surprising lands of India, is finally accepted in the West as worthy of being inserted into our habits.

After years of researching myself through the readings that made me the person I am today - as well as being open to the practice of personal growth and becoming a teacher myself - it took me years to understand the real power released by this word of only four letters.

Four letters, a whole world to discover.

Four letters, the possibility of opening ourselves to the great enlightenment inside and outside us.

You will have heard this word everywhere ... and therefore: what exactly is Yoga?

Yoga is a practice that recalls mind and body with a 5,000-year history that stems from ancient Indian philosophy. Different styles of Yoga combine meditation or relaxation techniques, physical postures, breathing, moral principles and healthy habits, and elements that make up - like strong and mighty branches - an ancient tree, full of wisdom and solidity.

The first important notion is to consider this word not only a physical practice (the so-called asanas, the prominent poses that are part of it) but a whole natural lifestyle with a millennial history that involves many aspects of our life ... This is why the first helpful concept is to understand what awaits you when you approach it during your 'senior days'.

In recent years, Yoga has become very popular as a pose-based workout that promotes control of the mind and body and improves internal and external balance and well-being. Yet, this is a limited vision of many teachings handed down first through orality by the yogi masters to the disciples and then thanks to the spread of the Upanishads and the Bhagavad Gita, two Indian written works in which this practice was named to arrive at the enlightenment of the soul.

In 500 BC, however, we can find the first work wholly dedicated to Yoga, exactly in Patanjali's Yoga Sutra, a collection of 196 aphorisms that narrate and hand down all the bases of the discipline. The Yoga Sutra is still today a guide on how to master the mind, control emotions, and grow spiritually.

Over the years, moreover, the writing has become the sacred text par excellence of Yoga, a reference point for anyone who wants to begin to understand it and understand what it is about.

So … what does that have to do with you anyway?

How chair Yoga can amplify your senior days?

Now that we have discovered how Yoga is an increasingly requested discipline for the construction of one's inner and body well-being, you may ask yourself: why should I approach this practice during my senior years?

By 2050, two billion people worldwide will be over 60, a 100% increase from 2020. Every person in every country in the world should have the opportunity to live a long and healthy life, and Yoga can help us in this regard.

Many people think of Yoga as an activity that improves balance and promotes flexibility. However, it is so much more. Yoga classes incorporate breathing, relaxation, and meditation exercises, increasing the individual's overall health and well-being.

That's why it is an ideal physical activity for seniors as it is low impact, can be modified with props and tools (even a comfy chair!) for different abilities, and can be started at any age.

Chapter 2
Chair Yoga for Seniors: Benefits

Physical benefits

So… Yoga for seniors can help solve or prevent several problems and enhance your well-being from each point of view.

The numerous benefits of Yoga are proven. Yoga is undeniable one of the best and most effective forms of exercise for seniors, as it has extensive benefits for their mental and physical health. These include:

- strengthening bones;
- reducing stress;
- improving sleep;
- decreasing physical pain;
- decreasing the risk of depression.

It also improves strength, flexibility, mobility, and balance, helping to avoid injuries. Let's find out all of them specifically.

Strengthening Bones and Muscles
Yoga helps prevent physiological changes, including osteopenia and sarcopenia, by strengthening bones and muscles. This is achieved by using and engaging the muscles and bones through the practice of Yoga.

Pain Relief
Regardless of your physical limitations, Yoga is excellent for reducing aches and pains from aging. In particular, people suffering from physiological changes, such as sarcopenia and osteopenia, can benefit greatly from Yoga by learning to breathe and relax properly to cope with chronic pain.

Reducing Stress

Several studies show that Yoga reduces cortisol levels, the main stress hormone in the brain. This greatly reduces stress and anxiety. Using Yoga alone or with other practices, such as meditation, is an excellent way to keep stress levels down. Additionally, Yoga can benefit those suffering from various types of anxiety disorders by helping to decrease people's anxiety levels.

Improving sleep

Sleep is often a problem for seniors for various reasons. The practice of Yoga for seniors offers relaxation that promotes longer and deeper sleep.

Reducing the risk of depression

Yoga is good for mood, just like the good mood pill for decreasing the chances of depression. It also lowers the levels of cortisol, the stress hormone. In that way, our body's serotonin levels increase, improving our overall happiness.

Improving Flexibility, Mobility, and Balance

Practicing Yoga helps increase balance and agility through slow, controlled poses. It empowers people to prevent falls, the leading cause of injury for the elderly.

N.B. Yoga practitioners over the age of 65 are at greater risk of injury than other age groups. If you are new to Yoga, chances are you will experience pain and soreness from using new muscles. While there are risks of injury, the likelihood is low in senior Yoga compared to higher-impact physical activities.

Nonetheless, I always recommend contacting your doctor or treating physician before engaging in any physical activity.

Mental benefits

Apart from the physical benefits, one of the best benefits of Yoga is related to the work it does on our mind.

I admit I have come to embrace this discipline attracted precisely by the benefits it has on the person's thoughts, especially in managing stress and intrusive thoughts, which is known to have devastating effects on the body and mind at any age.

And this is more true for those who suffer from the classic 'ailments' of age which, consequently, trigger very strong negative feelings in them (sense of guilt, isolation, depression, loss of hope, etc.).

Yet it is the mind that is primarily responsible for both our unhappiness and our happiness. And we must remember to train it constantly to see lasting benefits over time, just like we do with the body.

That is why, thanks to Chair Yoga and meditation, we can find an effective and fast method to insist on our constant work on the mind, thanks to a millenary discipline that is also born to give back to mind itself a space of love and compassion.

On the other hand, a hostile environment in our mind also spills over into the body, and vice versa. Stress can present itself in many ways, including back or neck pain, sleep problems, headaches, substance abuse, and an inability to concentrate in your daily tasks. And Yoga can be very effective in developing those coping skills you still lack and reaching a more positive vision of life. With collaboration between body, mind and soul you can live your years peacefully.

The incorporation of meditation and breathing into Yoga, therefore, can help improve a person's mental well-being. Exciting, don't you think?

The regular practice of Yoga on the mind, ultimately:

- Creates mental clarity and calm;
- Increases body awareness;
- Relieves chronic stress patterns;
- Relaxes your mind;
- Helps you focus the attention;
- Favors the early diagnosis of physical problems;
- Allows early preventive action and immediate resolution of highlighted physical problems.

Spiritual benefits

The incorporation of meditation and breathing into Yoga, as I have repeatedly stated, can help improve a person's mental well-being, which in turn has a virtuous impact on our relationship with ourselves.

Linked to the benefits on body and mind, Yoga also helps with its benefits for the soul... which in my opinion are even more essential for living our life fully and with gratitude. Using the correct pranayama breathing techniques and through the slow, meditative movements of many traditional Yoga exercises, therefore, you can slow the heart rate, calm the body and activate the parasympathetic nervous system - giving your Soul the contemplation time it needs to help the body to function at its best.

Yoga also heals inner wounds. Retirement, relationships with others, the partner, a body image that we do not recognize anymore... Yoga can be wonderful, therefore, precisely for the recovery of those feelings of peace and well-being that at an unconscious level crave.

The transformative power of Yoga, ultimately, acts at the level of the soul when we are able, through practice, to restore the order of priorities and to recover those passions that make us live every day by doing only 'what gives us real joy', to put it as the tidying guru Marie Kondo would say.

Yoga, as we have seen, is a weapon against depression. It has proven to be an effective complementary therapy for those suffering from depression. Not only the induced calm but the physical nature of many of the exercises, in fact, releases endorphins, giving a natural (albeit temporary) boost to mood.

Those who suffer from repetitive depressive thoughts, on the other hand, may find that traditional Yoga allows their psyche time to 'eliminate' such negative obsessive thought cycles, making the psyche fresher, more robust, and able to react to shocks (the famous 'resilience'!).

Finally, Yoga prevents mental illness. Recent studies are beginning to show that Yoga, far from being a simple healing tool, can actually be a preventative measure aimed at protecting people from the mental illnesses they may develop (where genetic predispositions exist). And this happens especially if you practice the discipline from an early age.

Those who develop the ability to harness the most transcendent qualities of Yoga early in life, therefore, are particularly well positioned to protect their psyche from the stresses and strains of modernity. A skill that, once acquired, can be used throughout life, especially in adulthood.

As I wrote previously, therefore, undertaking the practice of Yoga which incorporates the spiritual and physical aspects of the art, is, ultimately, immensely useful for living life to the fullest of our abilities.

It allows the mind to connect with its deepest self and gives the psyche the opportunity to heal or 'eliminate' those lacerations of the Soul and those worrying patterns of behavior that can lead to the development of many pathologies.

Chair Yoga: your wellness ally

An easy way to approach Yoga is doing some simple body awareness exercises that you can do while sitting in a chair.

• These chair yoga exercises can help you keep your spine mobile;
• They can also help you improve rib cage mobility;

- Plus, they can help improve body awareness, which is good because it means your muscles are still active;
- Some of the exercises and poses you will encounter in the following pages can also help fight back pain.

Perhaps the first thing that comes to your mind when you think of Chair Yoga is a group of seniors. Indeed, Chair Yoga can be suitable for people of advanced age.

However, what is 'old'? Some older people have excellent mobility and strength, allowing them to regularly attend yoga classes. Some young people, on the other hand, have health problems or limitations that prevent them from moving like other people their age. Therefore, remember that Chair Yoga is mainly aimed at people with minimal mobility.

So, what is the difference between Chair Yoga and regular yoga? A Chair Yoga session is different from a regular yoga routine in several ways:

- The class moves at a slower pace than formal lessons;
- The exercises are very delicate, putting a strain on the joints. The chair is used as a support, which is also of great help in case of balance problems;
- Many classic yoga asanas can be adapted to be included in a Chair Yoga workout;

Therefore, Chair Yoga offers a myriad of benefits you are willing to achieve during your senior years:

- Working to improve joint mobility and all range of motions;
- With regular practice, improving balance and coordination;
- By moving in different ways in the chair and simply bringing awareness to the body posture, Chair Yoga helps improve the body's overall stance;
- The different exercises positively affect blood circulation;
- By gently activating all muscles, Chair Yoga's simple and quick exercises promote overall strength and stability against aging and osteoporosis;
- Enduring inner calm and balance;
- Preserving youth;
- Preserving falling prevention;
- Managing bloating for menopause;
- Promoting inner balance, calm, and also a peaceful life ahead;
- Helping create a fun daily routine with your children and grandchildren!

Chapter 3
Chair Yoga Questions and Answers

How can I start doing Yoga at 50-60+ years old?

Here are some excellent tips and tricks to start your practice smoothly:

- Assess your physical condition before starting: some positions are not recommended for those with certain medical conditions. That's why speaking to your doctor before taking even a simple yoga class is advisable. Plus, this will help you decide which course is right for you and make sure it aligns with your goals.

- You need to get the proper yoga clothing. The practice of Yoga requires comfortable clothing and also a non-slip Yoga towel, an attractive complementary accessory if you sweat a lot. It is a towel the size of a mat that you can wash in a machine. I always recommend you have one.

- Choose the right tools: you will also need a yoga mat that is long enough for the whole body when you are lying down. This will guarantee you support during all yoga poses. There is a wide variety of options on the market, with different characteristics, thicknesses, and prices. Ideally, you should choose a non-slip yoga mat. This way, you will prevent your hands and feet from slipping on them. Even if we are using chairs, it is essential to have one of them so that you feel good practicing in contact with your yoga mat if you are willing to lay down. Moreover, to carry your mat and keep it protected and clean, I recommend carrying it in a closed bag.

- Support items: for those suffering from joint pain, such as knees or wrists, tools are available that provide additional cushion and support. Additionally, straps and locks can make challenging positions more accessible. Yoga blocks are an optional type of yoga material but are very useful for exploring new postures and bringing comfort to your practice, even for Chair Yoga. They are made of cork or foam. The standard size is a brick, but new shapes and sizes appear. The yoga strap is an accessory that can help people with little flexibility reach their feet. We will address this tool in the poses section.

- Zafu or meditation cushion: many people also ask me about meditation cushions. They are high and hard cushions that allow you to keep your back straight and upright, relax your hips without getting too tired. Although you can sit on one or several cushions, or on a yoga block to meditate, the zafu is the most comfortable option for your hips. The half-moon zafu allows hip vascularity and can be more comfortable because they allow hip vascularity forward. In any case, it is a matter of taste and preferences. Every body has needs.

- As you can't finish a class without a good Savasana or Chair Savasana :), choose one that covers your entire body. It is one of my favorite accessory.

- Be sure to seek out a qualified yoga instructor who understands the potential limitations and unique challenges that people aged 60 or older face. Once you've chosen your instructor, be sure to let them know if you have any health conditions, so you can proceed safely and efficiently. They will be able to help you find an exercise program that aligns with your goals and interests. Logically, the exercises in this book are simple and easy to understand, which you can do at home on your own. But you can always ask for confirmation of the right positions for you and the flows you can perform according to your health conditions.

- Try to start slowly and start with a light workout. Make yourself goals that you can achieve over time (for example, touching your toes). This way, you can focus on the correct technique and gradually improve with a low risk of injury. Yoga is not about comparing yourself with others but rather about moving and improving at your own pace. Although you may feel distressed, Yoga should never hurt or cause you pain. Remember that almost any position can be changed to suit your needs, and make sure you are comfortable.

Is Yoga good for seniors?

Yoga is one of the best forms of exercise for seniors. There are different types and styles of Yoga, making it suitable for anyone. Yoga practitioners have many physical and mental health benefits, including strengthening bones, reducing stress, improving sleep, decreasing pain, and reducing the risk of depression. It also improves strength, flexibility, mobility, and balance.

How frequently should I do Yoga?

A study published in the Journal of the American Geriatrics Society (December 2016) is the first to have analyzed the positive effects of Chair Yoga on people with osteoporosis and arthritis. The researchers conducted an experiment on a group of elderly people suffering from chronic osteoporosis. Some of them have been sent to follow a Chair Yoga program, consisting of two lessons a week of 45 minutes each. Other patients have instead followed a normal physical education course.

The scholars measured some parameters before, during, and after the sessions, such as pain, the latter's interference in daily life, the speed of gait, and the degree of fatigue. The results obtained show that the oriental discipline helps to decrease pain and falling, increase the speed of movements, and reduce fatigue.

Also the Journal of Human Kinetics, moreover, recently published a study showing that older women who practiced Yoga three times a week for twelve weeks experienced a significant improvement in their respiratory function.

So, to answer the question, a constant and daily practice of just 5-10 minutes can help you feel better and rediscover the pleasant sensations of lightness, happiness, and balance.

What kind of Yoga is best for seniors?

- Chair Yoga (of course!): it is considered a 'non-traditional' option for seniors who are not comfortable with up and down movements but are still interested in the benefits of Yoga. Chair yoga for seniors changes traditional postures, including standing postures, to be performed in a chair in a simple and effective way.

- Hatha Yoga: Hatha Yoga is a gentle form of Yoga that often consists of a series of standing and sitting postures that focus on stretching and breathing. This yoga sequence is believed to be the best for beginners.

- Restorative Yoga: Restorative Yoga is a slow, meditative form of Yoga that uses supportive objects to support the body while holding positions for long periods. This gentle sequence is one of the best form of Yoga for seniors who wish to achieve feelings of relaxation and satisfaction. We will address one powerful restorative flow in the following chapters!

- Yin Yoga: Yin Yoga is similar to Restorative Yoga as it focuses on slow movements. The main difference is that Yin Yoga focuses on stretching the deep connective tissue, helping to relieve stiffness while increasing flexibility.

- Ashtanga Yoga: Ashtanga Yoga is challenging and fast and combines a series of postures that are demonstrated in the same way every time. It uses flexibility and increases heart rate and circulation, making it excellent for weight loss. Ashtanga yoga is not recommended for beginners. However, many seniors could find it very useful.

- Kundalini Yoga: Kundalini Yoga combines postures, breathing exercises, meditation, and chants. It is an excellent course for older adults interested in more than the physical aspects of Yoga because it also uses spiritual components.

- Vinyasa Yoga: Vinyasa is a term that encompasses yoga styles that involve pairing breathing with a series of movements that flow together to create a fast, fluid routine. Vinyasa yoga classes vary in difficulty and are recommended for relatively fit seniors looking for a greater challenge.

Last but not least: what about the chair?

Since Chair Yoga's verb is "adaptability," it shouldn't be surprising that the home chair is perfect for practice. It is not important which chair you want to use. Any type is fine; the important thing is ... to practice!

Just make sure that it is a chair with a stable back and, if your balance allows it, without handles ... also because for some positions, you will see, these could be uncomfortable and not allow you to perform the exercises correctly.

The only limitations are chairs with any wheels, or office chairs, as they often turn out to be unstable. In this case, there must be a special block on the wheels or a mat that causes friction.

Chapter 4
Chair Yoga: False Myths

Let's face it: despite Yoga, its discipline and practice have now become widespread among many people, there are still some clichés that must be debunked.

In particular, in this section, we will try to address the 'false myths' mainly related to the practice of Yoga through asanas and physical postures.

Thinness

This myth goes something like this: only thin people can do Yoga. Nothing more false! Yoga is a universal discipline, and everyone can practice it: from the child to the elderly, from the fit person to the one with physical problems, and, therefore, those who have a few extra pounds!

In addition to being a consideration dictated by the lack of knowledge of the discipline itself, thinking the opposite does not take into account its enormous power in transforming the body one step at a time. One of the main objectives of Yoga is precisely to restore balance to the body by connecting with it at a deep level. And that there are a few difficulties between our thoughts, our soul, and our chakras do not matter at all!

Indeed, through Yoga, you will regain your strength and balance by increasing confidence and muscle mass without retracing the old paths that have not helped you until now.

Perfection

I admit it: at first, I also thought that to be a good and disciplined Yoga student, I had to become perfect, which meant precisely replicating the teacher's positions.

Well, precisely through constant practice - both alone and in groups - I understood not only that every body is different and that each one has its own intrinsic 'limits' dictated by the composition, but also that it is much more useful to focus on the benefits than on the 'Olympic' execution.

On the other hand, many styles of Yoga do not aspire to perfection (except in some ways Iyengar Yoga) but rather to the fluidity of movements dictated by how flexible and strong we have become through daily practice. Put simply: fluency always beats perfection!

Flexibility

'If I am not flexible, I cannot do Yoga.' Once again, a comment dictated by the fact that, perhaps, we have never tried to move the body using Yoga in support.
It is not necessary that you manage to do the most difficult or complex positions when you start, also because there are always simplified variations that have the SAME EFFECT of the most challenging ones.
On the other hand, sometimes flexibility isn't even an advantage! When you are too flexible, you have a greater tendency to extend the ligaments that were not created to get up to that point, which could also hurt in the long run.

Age

Here we are! As we have seen refuting the thesis of Thinness, age is also a real false myth. Many people think that after 'a certain age,' doing Yoga would be impossible if not harmful.
All this is just a condition of thought dictated by the concept that an aging person could get injured in the bones and muscles. That it would be, in practice, 'dangerous' for some to do Yoga.
Yet, Yoga is not only very safe if performed with simplicity but also very, very useful for preventing precisely that muscle and bone aging caused by too much sedentary lifestyle or advancing age.
As with the mind, training the body by starting slowly and continuing steadily can help people older in age to recover movements and a connection with them often forgotten.

Chapter 5
Meeting the Asanas

Asanas (Yoga poses) have become so popular worldwide that they are confused with the entire Yoga discipline because they are a useful and practicable tool for anyone to start the journey. It is unthinkable in our society, with all the stimuli to which we are constantly subjected, with the adverse culture that permeates us, to think of acting directly on the mind to appease its distractions.

It is also difficult to start the journey by trying to change habits: this is a society raised to be habitual. Since school, many children out of line, instead of being considered healthy and full of will to live, are punished, frustrated, or made to take medicines to get them back into the ranks. Likewise, in the world of work, we are subjected to strict hierarchies which we are bound to obey. Otherwise, they make us feel stupid, wrong, or incapable. And finally, during the senior years, seniors are completely marginalized by a narrative that does not consider them active in society. We are not surprised, therefore, if a large portion of the adult world population takes psychiatric drugs daily.

However, there is an instrument that looks like gymnastics and that works underneath to radically change our lives: this instrument is the asana. It starts like this: after some time, we feel better, both physically and mentally, and we have that much more energy that can be spent to start taking control of our life.

Asanas are practiced to promote good health and make the body stable and flexible to prepare it for pranayama and meditation.

The practice of the asanas itself, however, becomes a meditative act in itself when awareness is brought to the union between the body and the breath.

For this reason, even when it is fluid, the sequence of poses must be performed slowly - as long as it is not aimed at specific therapeutic purposes. While relying on the control of the limbs and muscles, it is more energetic than muscular work, aimed at awakening, together with other techniques, the power of kundalini, or dormant karmic energy.

The ultimate goal is to slow down movements, lengthening the breath to channel prana (or vital energy) towards a balance between opposing forces: stretching and compression, stabilization and extension, and potential and dynamic energy.

How are the asanas performed?

Asanas must be practiced with awareness, concentration, and control. An asana is performed from bottom to top following four actions:
- foundations;
- alignment;
- stabilization;
- extension.

It starts by establishing the foundations, that is, the parts in contact with the earth, and then arranging the body according to the universal principles of alignment. The correct alignment of an asana will favor its execution, but it is important to respect the constitution, personal abilities, and physical conformation in full respect of the functional anatomy.

The asanas must be stable and comfortable

It is important, in fact, to stabilize the center of gravity by activating the deep abdominals before stretching, extending, and expanding. The act of extension allows the full expression of a posture and the possibility of ultimately experiencing a state of absorption, lightness, and ease. The lengthening of the spine allows lateral, backward, or forward bending to occur organically, without effort.
Finally, how you enter and exit an asana is as important as the time you remain in the asana itself, not only to avoid injury but also to experience the practice as a meditation in motion.

How long do I have to hold a position?

Observe the breath: the quality of the breath indicates the duration of an asana. When it gets short, it's time to stop, catch up and change asanas. However, it is important to give the body time to respond.
A heated practitioner should remain in the posture for at least one minute to awaken the structural and physiological body. Beginners, however, shouldn't stay more than three deep breaths. It is advisable, perhaps, to repeat the same asana two or three times in a row.

How many asanas are there?

There are said to be 8 million asanas, as many as there are varieties of human beings. However, the best-known asanas are about thirty, of different levels. There are also several variations, modifications, and preparations. After all, there is a limit to the directions in which a human body can be arranged! We will see them all in the following section!

Chapter 6
Chair Yoga Asanas

To begin to understand the importance of alignment in yoga, especially for beginners, you can devote yourself to the practice of specific positions. Their simple execution provides the basics of good alignment and then refines and develops it even more with intermediate asanas, later more complex.

Basic asanas to familiarize yourself with yogic alignment are:

- Savasana (Corpse Pose) - Pg. 43-45

Intermediate asanas to familiarize yourself with yogic alignment are:

- Bhujangasana (Cobra Pose) - Pg. 46
- Trikonasana (Triangle Pose) - Pg. 47
- Utthita Parsvakonasana (Extended Side Angle)- Pg. 48
- Navasana (Boat Pose) - Pg. 49
- High Altar - Pg. 50
- Spinal Twists - Pg. 51
- Virabhadrasana I, II, III (Warrior Poses)
     - Virabhadrasana I - Pg. 52
     - Virabhadrasana II - Pg. 53
     - Virabhadrasana III - Pg. 54
- Viparita Virabhadrasana II (Reverse Warrior II Pose) - Pg. 55
- Ardha Kapotasana (Seated Pigeon Pose) - Pg. 56
- Garudasana (Eagle Pose) - Pg. 57

For each of the positions, we will also remember the original name in Sanskrit for knowledge and also so as not to get confused with their names when you hear them from a video, from a teacher, or from a yogic companion.

Obviously, for each of the positions, we will show the chair variant, taking care to remember that this type of Yoga does not and will never detract from the benefits and effectiveness of each single 'classic' Yoga pose.

You will also find some flows, or sequences of poses, dedicated to some memorable moments for your practice, while in Book 7, 'Workout for Well-Being,' you can discover all the main flows for Wellness that also include the aid of such a discipline as powerful as the Yoga Chair!

Good discovery, enjoy these practices... and Namasté!

Chapter 7
Go with the Flow

Warm up and breathing

What differentiates an asana from a simple gymnastic exercise is precisely the attention to the breath. It is, in fact, the breath that sets the movement and guides the practice.

In general, you inhale in the stretches and exhale every time you create compression on the abdomen. All asanas, however, can be performed without risk while exhaling.

Many people think that the correct way to breathe is to inhale through the nose and exhale through the mouth. It is not so.

However, for now, assume that correct breathing must always be done through the nose, also because the techniques of breathing from the mouth are an overwhelming minority when compared to those in which the nose is used.

Mastery in the execution of an asana is indicated by the quality of the breath, which must be fair, deep, and slow.

In back and side bends, or when the effort is required, breathing becomes shorter - and that's normal. It is important, however, never to remain in apnea while performing an asana. You always breathe through the nose to have greater control of the respiratory flow. To start, try some adapted and easy breathing exercises.

Although breathing is automatic and uncontrolled is a function that we take for granted; listening to ourselves, gradually becoming aware of the way we breathe, and trying to exercise control over the breath allows us to understand if we are relaxed and mentally calm.

In general, you must enter the pose with the right breath. That's how:

• Push-ups or forward bends (e.g.: Uttanasana): EXPIRATION
• Push-ups or back bends and expansions (e.g.: Bhunjangasana): INSPIRATION
• Lateral push-ups or push-ups (e.g., Utthita Trikonasana): INSPIRATION
• Twists or rotations of the body (e.g.: Parivrtta Trikonasana): EXPIRATION

In general, try to adopt this pattern for all the positions you perform. I know very well that initially it is not easy but, thanks to constant practice, you will be able to enter the positions in the correct way.

This previous scheme will help you when taking an asana.

Asana flow = pose sequence

The word 'Flow,' in addition to 'yoga,' is inspired by Vinyasa Yoga, one of the many interpretations of the ancient Indian discipline. It is dynamic yoga in which the asanas (positions) flow in a coordinated sequence marked by the rhythm of the breath.

Yoga flow, therefore, allows you to synchronize breath and movement, combining a series of postures (asanas) in a single flow.

The main feature, therefore, of this discipline is the fluidity of the movements while keeping the attention on breathing for the entire duration of the session.

Hence, after having warmed up the body through correct breathing (which we will see later when we will show the poses), the next step in any yoga practice is to choose a sequential composition of asanas, called flow.

We will dedicate the last part of the book to the execution of different Yoga flows, without prejudice to learning every single pose to perfection.

Final relaxation

The final relaxation allows you to completely regenerate and free your mind in just a few minutes.

Through this moment, with your eyes closed and in a completely relaxed position, you will allow the body to absorb what it has just done for you.

You will be able to feel immense gratitude for having granted you the benefits of the practice and to listen to all the tension points on which to direct attention, even given the next practice.

That is why I always recommend never skipping the final relaxation (in most cases in the Savasana pose), even if it were only a couple of minutes.

Chapter 8
Beginner Poses

UJJAYI BREATHING (VICTORIOUS / OCEAN BREATHING)

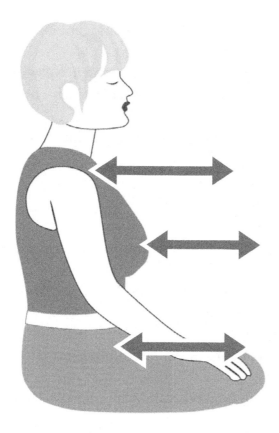

It is a breathing technique used to calm the mind and warm the body.

When practicing Ujjayi, one begins to fill the lungs with air by breathing through the nose and maintaining a slight throat contraction.
It is often used during the practice of vinyasa and ashtanga yoga. When done correctly, the whispering sound has given this breathing the name of ocean breath.

To perform it, inhale and then exhale with your mouth closed, through your throat. It will be familiar with some practice. Be careful not to close your throat. You will repeat this for several breaths.

This technique will teach you to control your breathing, one of the essential parts of yoga. It will also help you live in the present moment by connecting your mind, body, and spirit, calming the mind, releasing tensions, and any accumulation of emotions.

If it is your first time trying this breathing exercise, you should do it with a certified instructor to guide you. Stop the procedure if you feel dizzy.
If you have any health problems, consult a doctor first.

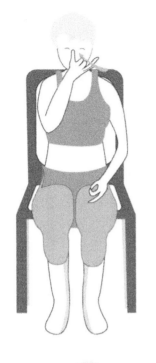

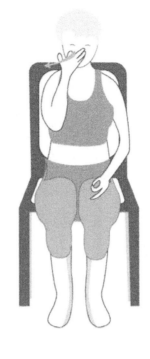

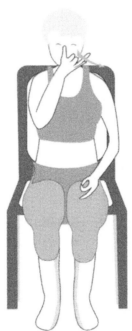

Place your left hand on your thigh; with the right hand, place the index and middle fingers on the forehead, in the space between the two eyebrows, and place the thumb on the right nostril and the ring finger on the left nostril.

Inhale from the right nostril for a few seconds, closing the left nostril with the ring finger.

Hold your breath for 4 seconds, and then blocking the right nostril with your thumb, exhale from the left nostril that you left free from the ring finger.

Do the same reverse procedure: inhale from the left nostril blocking the right, hold for a few seconds and then exhale from the right nostril blocking the left; then go on alternating your breathing for a few minutes.

NECK RELEASE

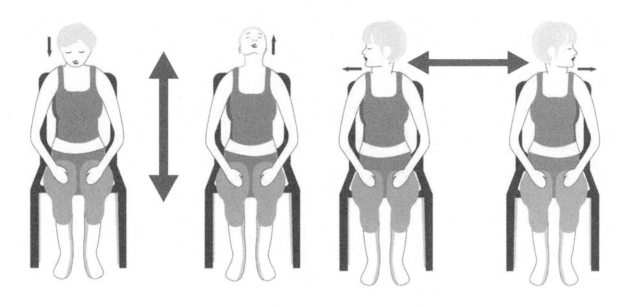

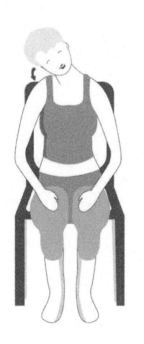
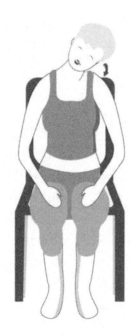

One of the first Chair Yoga poses that you will master is one of the most important for your well-being.

Starts by sitting straight, with your shoulders down, your neck muscles relaxed, and hands on your knees.
You will need to move your head in coordination with your breath.

Look up and go back to the center; look down and go back to the center. Then look towards the right and left shoulder and finally bring your ear to one shoulder and the other.

Close the pose with a neck circle, first clockwise and then counterclockwise. Move slowly, slower than you would, and open your eyes to prevent dizziness.

SHOULDER RELEASE

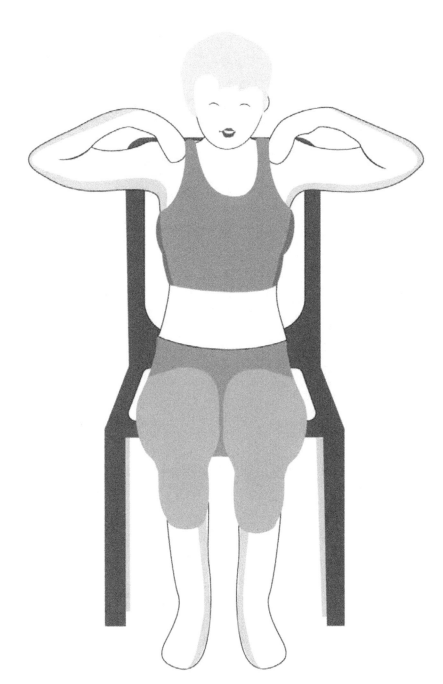

Moving the shoulders is essential to promote mobility and warm up the body before the practice.

Sit straight with your chest open and your feet firmly on the floor.

Then slowly, move your shoulders up and down, back and forth, and then proceed with backward rotations.

Breathing from the abdomen with each movement is vital to relax the muscles and prepare us for our practice.

You can use slow exhalations, counting 4 to inhale and 8 to exhale. Gradually increase the number of exhalations to 12 and 16.
This has an immediate calming effect on the nervous system.

HIP RELEASE

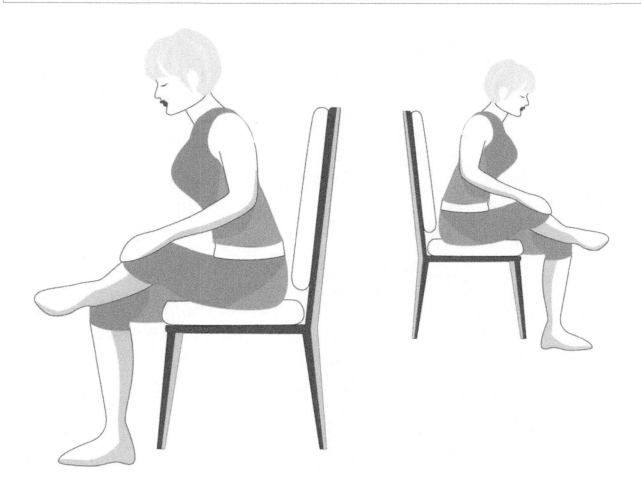

This exercise is great for relieving tension in the hips and lower back and irritation of the sciatic nerve.

Start by sitting forward, towards the edge of the chair. Place the right heel on the left knee in a 'four' position. The knee will fall to the right side.

Continue gently bending forward until you feel a stretch in your right hip joint. To deepen, gently press the knee down with the elbows. If there is tension or pressure in the knee, back off a little. For maximum benefit, repeat the pose a second time before continuing.

Make sure to repeat the same sequence on the other side.

KNEE RELEASE

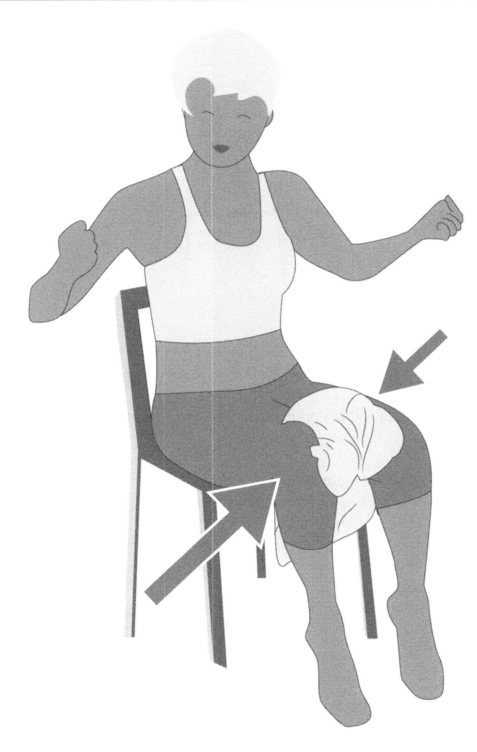

Knee discomfort is a common complaint in aging populations. As we age, it is very important to develop strength around the knee joint by performing exercises like these.

Start by placing a thin but firm pillow between your knees and bring your feet together. Sit straight and keep your legs at a 90-degree angle.

Press your knees strongly together, squeezing the pillow while breathing. Hold for 15 to 20 seconds.

Then repeat 3 to 5 times.

Make sure to repeat the same sequence on the other side.

ANKLE RELEASE

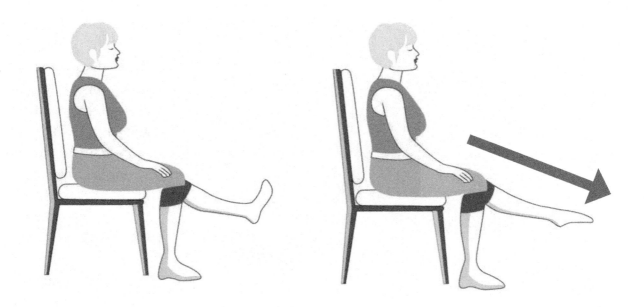

We often underestimate the mobility and strength of our feet, but this is a key factor in maintaining mobility and independence as we age. These exercises can help.

Sit well with your back straight and resting on the backrest and your feet firmly on the ground.

Raise your right leg without exaggerating and start to rotate the ankle clockwise at least five times; stop and make another five rotations counterclockwise.

Place your feet back on the ground and lift your left leg, repeating the rotation with the left ankle first in one direction and then in the other. Return the leg to the starting position and take a few breaths to rest.

Do this at least three/ four times per leg.

HAMSTRING STRETCH WITH BELT

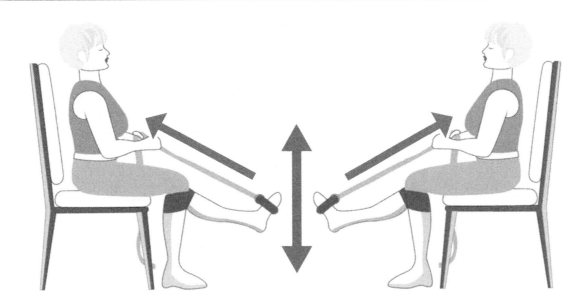

The use of this tool does not have the purpose of intensifying a position in an unnatural way or of anticipating the times of the body: it must be seen as a support, an accompaniment. Listening to yourself is, as always, the best way to understand if these tools are for us or if it is better, in our practice, to leave them in the bag.

The belt can be used for forwarding bends, but while seated. In fact, if our back is not sufficiently loose to allow us to touch our feet with our hands, then it, passed around the feet and taken with the hands, will allow us to hold the position more comfortably.

Sit in the usual starting position and gently tie a knot in the belt, neither too big nor small: it will have to naturally contain your foot.

Place the knot of the belt under the sole of the right foot and, always gently, pull the belt towards you to help you slowly stretch your leg until you reach the height that is feasible for you.

Better not to overdo it, especially at the beginning: slowly, with consistency, this simple exercise will support you in greater joint flexibility. Always remember to inhale and exhale and to relax the shoulders and face muscles.

Repeat everything in the second leg.

PALMS ON BELLY (SUKHASANA BELLY POSE)

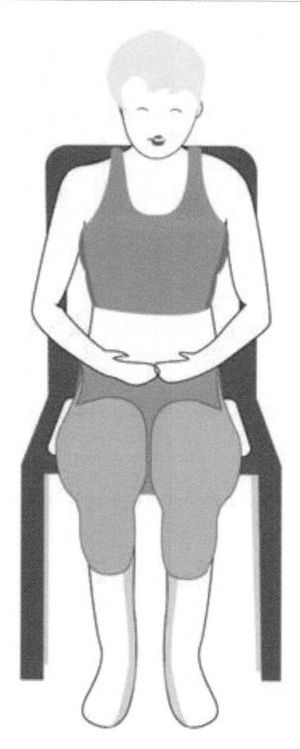

Even if you are not an expert, learning the Sukhasana position opens your perception to a state of inner awareness (the door to meditation).

You will notice a small but consistent change in thinking, no longer so hyper-kinetic and active; rather a feeling of 'centering' and stability.

After becoming aware of the alignments, watch the breath expand and feel the movements of the muscles of the eyes, the jaw, and the tongue settle into a sweet smile.

To perform this pose, stand still with your feet planted on the ground.

And then put your hands on your stomach, inserting inhalations and exhalations of equal length.

Closes your eyes and breath for 4-5 cycles of inhale/exhale.

TADASANA (MOUNTAIN POSE)

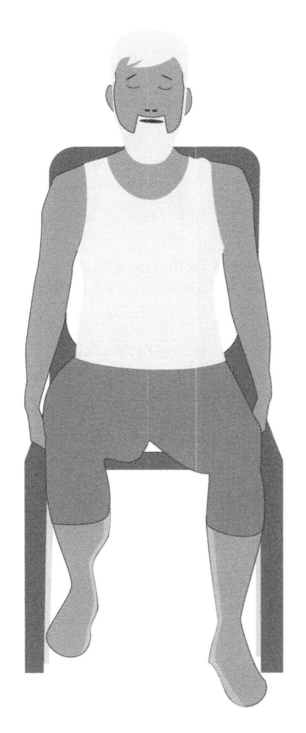

This pose helps to stretch the spine, stretch the back muscles and energize the body.

Start by sitting high at the end of the chair.

Stretch the chest, shoulders, and arms upwards as much as possible.

Keep your palms and fingers relaxed, not tense, nor rigid.

Relax your shoulder muscles, stretch your neck and keep it aligned with your spine.

This is the final position.

Maintain it as long as you can sustain the effort in a balanced way, breathing normally.

MARJARYASANA / BITILASANA (CAT & COW SEQUENCE)

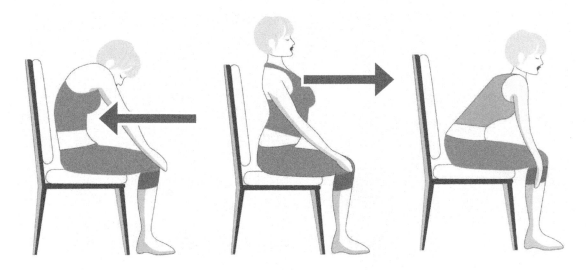

The Cat and Cow Pose is a classic yoga pose that helps build the connection between the lower spine and pelvis, as well as the upper spine and shoulders. Fortunately, it can easily be done in a chair!

Sit on the chair with both feet flat on the floor. Sit close to the edge of the chair.

Put your hands on your knees or on the top of your thighs. Breathe in.

During an inhalation, slowly arch your back, bringing your chest forward and pulling your tailbone and shoulders back (Cow pose).

Then arch the spine by pushing the chest out and as you exhale forcefully, bring the shoulders back to their place and continue like this (Cat pose). Inhale and exhale as you arch your torso downwards.

To exhale, around the back, pulling the chest back and pulling the tailbone and shoulders forward.

Repeat 3 to 5 times.

HANDS TO THE CHEST (ANJALI MUDRA)

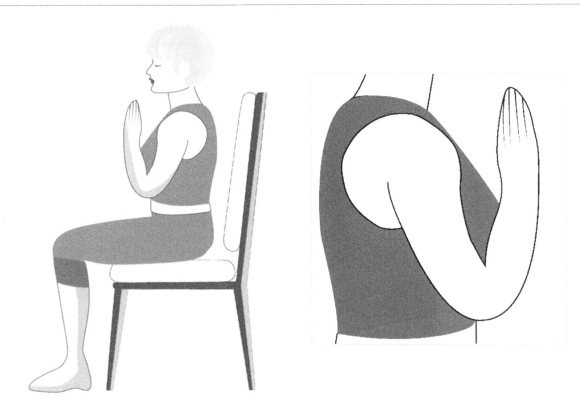

Mudras are shapes that we give to our hands, points of power in the fingers, seals of ancient origin, actually used all over the world, not only in India. We think about our daily life, about crossing our fingers, clapping our hands, shaking them to introduce ourselves, and as a sign of greeting. These are also powerful gestures.

How to practice Anjali mudra?

We join our palms at our hearts, fingers touching but leaving a small space between the palms. Then we inhale and exhale normally for 2-3 breaths.

The pressure of the fingers must always be light and give us a pleasant feeling; the hands must not be tense or rigid but loose. This is because, between palm and palm, we want to let the energy of our body flow.

Urdhva Hastasana (Raised Hands Pose)

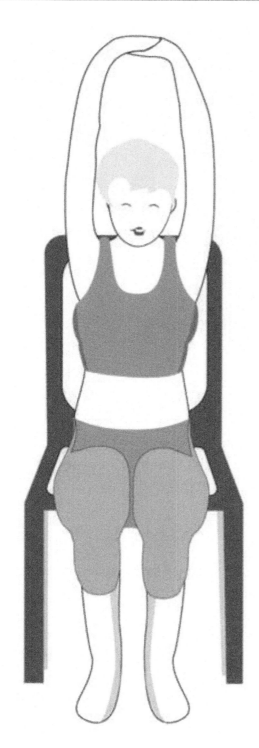

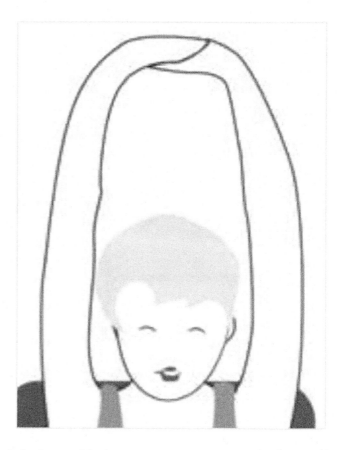

Inhale and bring your arms towards the ceiling. You can decide whether to keep your hands open at the same distance as the shoulders and arms or whether to join the palms.

Let the shoulder blades slide behind the back, which stretches upwards.

Stretch the muscles as much as you can, staying well anchored in the chair, after which exhale and return to the starting position.

APANASANA (KNEE TO CHEST POSE)

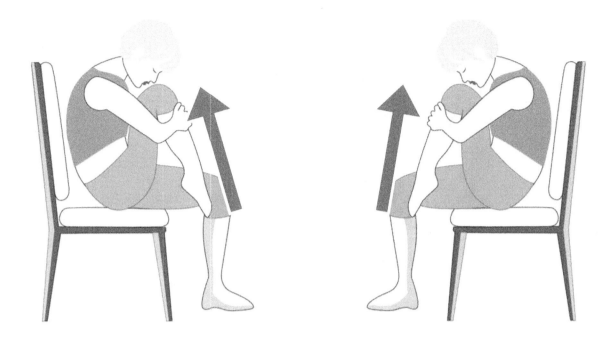

This is an excellent pose for relaxing the back and tense muscles of the neck and thighs.

All you have to do is sit on the chair and place your palms on your knees. Breathe in.

As you exhale, gently bring your legs closer to your chest, and as you inhale, release your grip and let your legs move completely away from your belly.

Do this exercise for a few minutes at your own pace, then let your breath guide your movements.

Maintain this position for some time and close your eyes; if your mind is not at rest, try counting your breaths.

This helps to calm the mind, and when you feel calm, slowly lower your legs to the floor and relax into the starting position.

UTTANANASA AND ARDHA UTTANANASA (FORWARD FOLD)

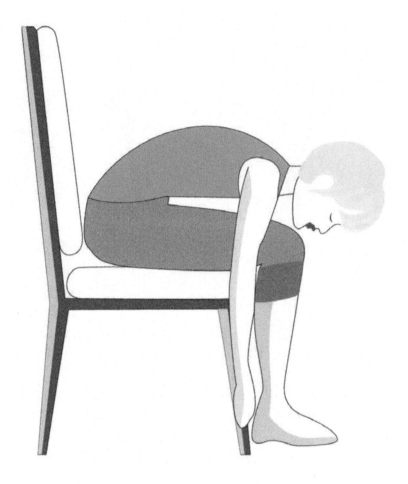

Inhale and raise your arms.

As you exhale, lean forward, resting your torso on your thighs.

If possible, place your hands on the floor and dangle your head. Rest in this position for a few breaths.

To exit, straighten your arms in front of you above your head and come up.

Repeat three times in total, and the last time you bend forward, stay there.

FORWARD FOLD VARIANT: RAGDOLL

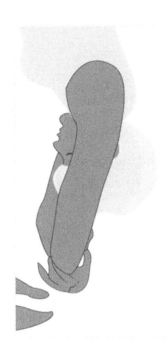

This position is called the 'ragdoll' because you will stretch and relax your neck, shoulders, and back going to bend forward. Just like a rag doll. So, here's how to do it.

Start by sitting down, keeping the back very straight and the legs apart from one another, a little wider than the hips.

Lean forward little by little. Then let yourself fall and relax your head, shoulders, and arms that you will let dangle. Tilt as much as you can but without forcing the position, and in the meantime, continue to inhale deeply.

Hold the position for 3-4 breaths and then slowly begin to rise with the back vertebra after vertebra. The head comes last.

While sitting, take a few breaths and then repeat.

FORWARD FOLD VARIANT: FORWARD BEND

Another variation of this pose is a standing one called 'forward bend', another great way to stretch your hamstrings and prevent hip and lower back pain!
This time we stand.

Place both hands on the shoulder-width backrest and walk back slightly until the torso begins to bend towards the floor. Maintain a slight bend in your knees and keep your back very straight as you bend forward.

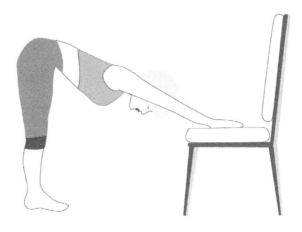

Inhaling, press the chair and return to an upright position.

SUKHASANA CACTUS ARMS POSE

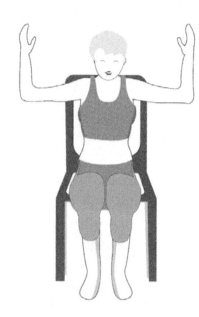

A simple position but capable of giving tone, strength, and energy to the body and arms.

Start in a sitting position, with your back resting on the back of the chair, your legs touching, and your feet firmly planted on the ground.

Then slowly raise your arms by bending your elbows to form a right angle with your body, to look a bit like a giant cactus.

Hold the position for 3-4 inhalation and exhalation cycles. Then lower your arms.

SUKHASANA (SIDE BEND VARIATION)

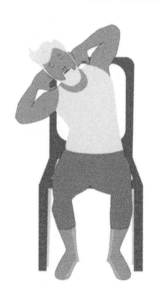 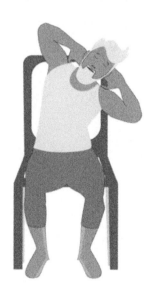

A variant from the Cactus Pose.

Start in a sitting position, with your back resting on the back of the chair, your legs touching, and your feet firmly planted on the ground.

Then slowly raise your arms by bending your elbows to form a right angle with your body, to look a bit like a giant cactus.

If you want to add the variation, then, before lowering the arms as in the previous exercise, you can keep the arms and slowly bend first to the left and then to the right.

Hold the position for 3-4 inhalation and exhalation cycles. And then lower your arms.

BADDHA KONASANA (BUTTERFLY POSE)

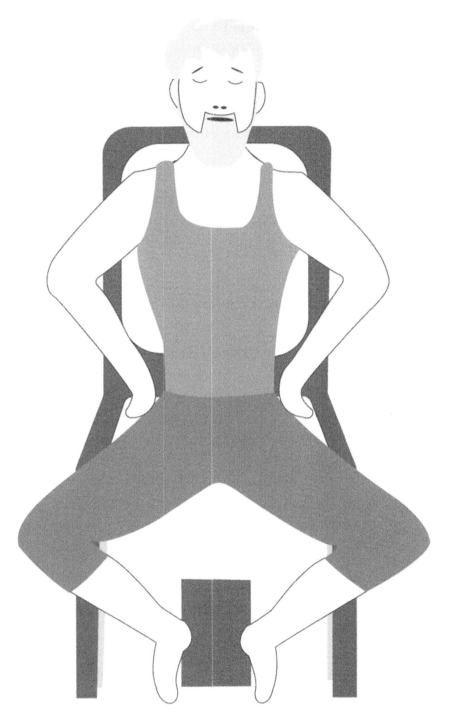

Butterfly Pose can be challenging for many bodies. So, if for some reason you can't practice, you can try this variation using your chair and your footing blocks.

Take your yoga blocks before sitting down. Then place them in the highest, vertical length and place your feet on top slowly.

The soles of the feet touch, while the knees fall sideways.

Don't force the opening: let gravity help you!

Bring your hands clasped to your hips, maintaining the position, and inhale and exhale for 3-5 breaths.

UTKATASANA (CHAIR POSE)

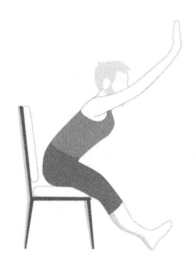

Although this position is born standing, like many other classic and basic Yoga positions, it is also very effective when seated.

The starting position for performing Utkatasana is Tadasana, the yoga posture of the Mountain.

As you inhale, raise your arms so that they are parallel to each other. Alternatively, you can close your palms.

As you exhale, bring your torso down, keeping it slightly bent forward.

Hold this position for 3-5 inhalation and exhalation cycles.

UTKATA KONASANA (GODDESS POSE)

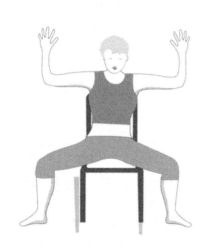

This yoga pose stretches the quadriceps, hamstrings, knees and ankles, thereby strengthening the different parts of the lower body, also helping relieve the symptoms of arthritis.

Start from the position of Tadasana, the Mountain Pose. Spread your legs one step and rotate your toes outwards. Pull your belly in so that you feel the back of your pelvis slightly forward.

Keep the knees in the line above the ankles to form a right angle.

Keep your torso erect and your abs active to keep your back in line. Raise your arms, bringing your elbows to shoulder height.

Stay in this position for a couple of breaths and push the tailbone forward, trying to stretch your back while keeping it straight.

VRKSASANA (TREE POSE)

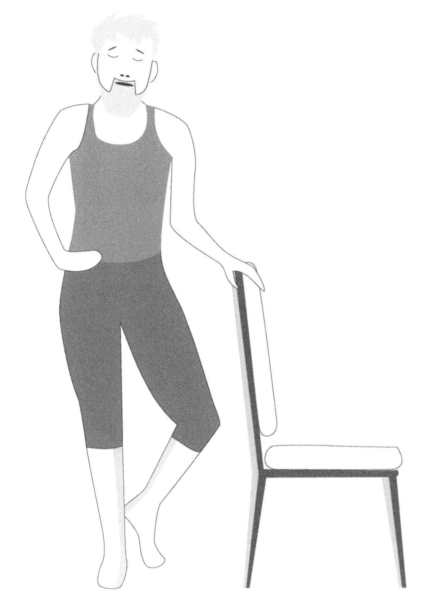

The Tree position is an excellent balance position for the elderly. We performe it standing, supported by the chair.

Place one foot on the opposite inner thigh (or lower). The leg should be turned to the side, with one hand positioned on the chair.

Hold this position for 5-8 breaths.

This position is suitable for older adults who risk suffering from hip pain and other problems. It increases the mobility of the hip and activates the muscles of the legs and abdominals, promoting balance and concentration.

The tree position requires firm abdominal muscles and also a good balance. And that is a problem for many seniors whose muscles are weakening and at risk of falling and injuring themselves.

So, if you are a beginner, you can also perform the tree pose on the wall with a chair, supporting the raised leg and leaning the rest of the body against the wall.

ADHO MUKHA SVANASANA (DOWNWARD FACING DOG)

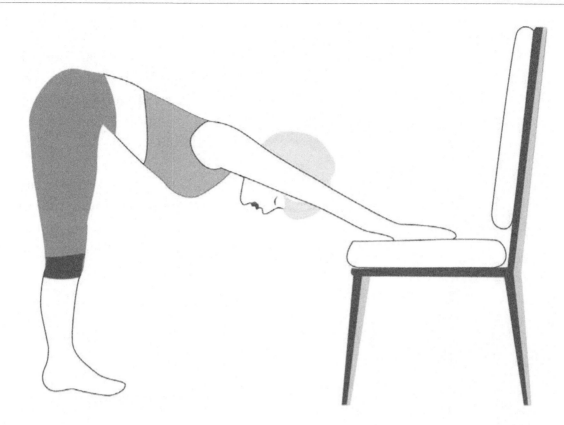

It is one of the most famous postures in yoga: it invigorates energy and is physically very demanding on the upper body. It strengthens the arms, shoulders, and abdomen muscles while also stretching the spine and hamstrings.

This pose also tones the digestive organs, also relieving headaches and menstrual discomfort. Especially if performed on a chair! Here's how to do it.

There are several variations for this position in Chair Yoga, which are very useful for those with sensitive wrists, upper body weakness, headaches, dizziness, or even balance problems.

Place both hands on the shoulder-width backrest and walk back slightly until the torso begins to bend towards the floor. Maintain a slight bend in your knees and keep your back very straight as you bend forward. Inhaling, press the chair and return to an upright position.

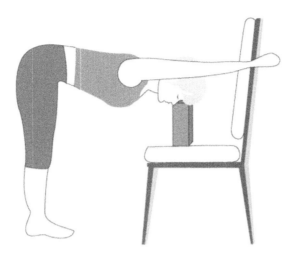

This one is a great way to stretch your hamstrings and prevent hip and lower back pain, allowing more than one stretch of the upper body.

This time we will use the chair but also a block, not to press too far with the bend.

Place both hands on the shoulder-width backrest and walk back slightly until the torso begins to bend towards the floor.

Make sure to maintain a slight bend in your knees. Also keep your back very straight as you bend forward. Keep some weight on the chair for support.

As you inhale, press into the back of the chair and return to an upright position.

SAVASANA (CORPSE POSE)

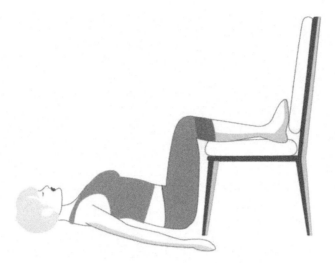

Although it sounds easy, the Corpse Pose (Savasana) is considered the most difficult of the asanas. In fact, many yoga students who can safely balance and do pushups and twists during class have a hard time lying on the floor.

That's why Savasana is a precious gift. The position creates the conditions for you to gradually enter a state of deep relaxation, which is extremely regenerating and an excellent starting point for meditation.

By resting your calves on support, you relax your legs, which can be fatigued by practicing yoga, exercising, and long hours spent standing or sitting. This variant also improves circulation and relieves tension in the back muscles, allowing you to achieve deeper relaxation.

On the other hand, raising the back and supporting the head helps open the chest, let go of the shoulders, and improve the natural flow of breath. If you are low on energy, low in spirits, or have a lot of tension in your upper back and shoulders, this variant is for you.

Perform a mental scan of the body from head to toe, gradually releasing each part of the body and each muscle group. Take the time to notice which points on your body come into contact with the floor. With each exhalation, imagine that each limb becomes heavier and heavier and stretches out a little more. Use supports to release pressure, release tension and relax completely.

Gradually, you will notice that a feeling of complete stillness draws you inwards, and your breathing becomes quiet, almost imperceptible.

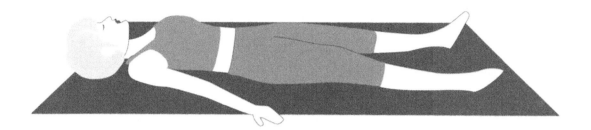

Place the mat in front of a chair or sofa.

Lie down in the center of the mat with your knees bent.

Raise your legs and place the back of your calves on the chair or sofa.

Rest the back of your arms on the floor with your palms facing up.

Arrange the support so that the entire calf, from the back of the knee to the heel, is evenly supported. If so, place a blanket under your head and neck (up to your shoulders) to lower your chin and direct your gaze down. If you wear glasses, take them off. If you want, place a cloth over your eyes. Rotate the upper arms to stretch the chest and, to raise the center, push the shoulder blades inside the back. The arms do not touch the torso at any point.

Relax your back muscles to spread out from the center to the sides. Bring attention to the entire back, feeling the rear ribs in contact with the floor. With each inhalation, the posterior ribs widen, and the lungs fill. With each exhalation, they contract. Try to feel the contact with the floor with all parts of the back, from the pelvis to the head.

CORPSE POSE: VARIANT 2

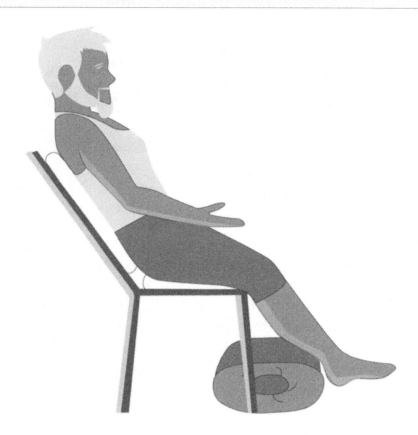

Sit on the chair with your back flat and your pelvis slightly forward.

Extend your legs forward, almost as an extension of the rest of your body, with your feet relaxed and your heels touching the ground.

Bring your hands to your belly, with your shoulders completely relaxed. Relax the muscles of the neck, face, and mouth. Breathe naturally.

Now close your eyes and bring your attention to your breath. Focus on filling your lungs evenly, right and left for a few minutes. Consciously expand the chest upwards and outwards as you inhale; release your breath.

Breath slowly. The practice of conscious breathing, through support, will have a calming effect on the nervous system.

Chapter 9
Intermediate Poses

BHUJANGASANA (COBRA POSE)

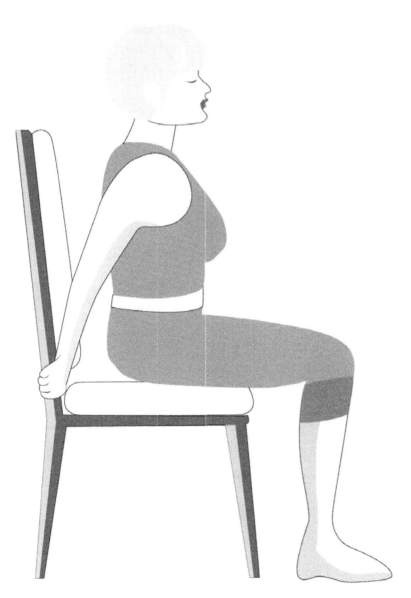

This exercise can help compensate for back slack during periods of prolonged sitting.

Start by sitting on the edge of the chair with your legs 90 degrees.

Hold the back of the chair with your arms straight, opening your chest and pushing it forward.
Expand across the front of your body, lifting your chin without throwing your head back. Let the spine gently arch.

Be careful; if there is any pinch or spasm in the back, back off slightly or release the pose and try again later.

Don't hold your breath while you are pushing forward.

TRIKONASANA (TRIANGLE POSE)

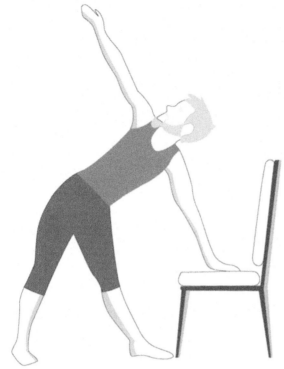

Trikonasana is a polar position; that is, it works on the two energetic aspects of the body: the yin, feminine, lunar, and the yang, masculine, solar. It's vital to keep these two aspects balanced (both from a physical and energetic point of view) to perform the position for the same duration on both sides.

This posture is one of the most complete because it contains a beautiful elongation of the body and an opening of the chest and hips, as well as being a balance asana.

In the variant with the chair, you enter this position while standing, opening the legs well as in the position of the Goddess.

One foot rotates to the side, and the other remains turned forward, with the external cut parallel to the chair, and the heels remain in the same straight line.

The arms open parallel to the floor, and the torso first moves parallel to the floor towards the rotated foot, then descends downwards to bring the hand towards the foot or to the ground.

The opposite part of the body stretches well; the arm rises upwards as if to insert the fingers of the hand into the ceiling, the chest rotates slightly outwards, and the gaze is directed towards the hand that is at the top.

In Trikonasana, the hips open to allow the pelvis to soften and the thighs to rotate outwards, while the well-held abdomen allows the torso not to slump forward but to maintain a nice straight and strong posture.

It is great for this position to use a chair that is not too high.

Utthita Parsvakonasana (Extended Side Angle)

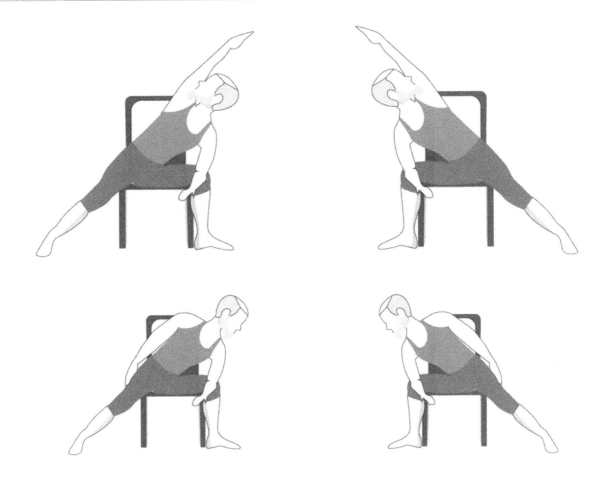

In your yoga practice is also important to perform a lateral stretch in order to access the full range of motion of the spine.

Sit on the edge of the chair. Spread your knees as far as possible, at a 90-degree angle if possible.

Place the right forearm on the top of the right thigh and gently press into the thigh.

Reach your left arm above your head; then start reaching the right side of the room, stretching the whole left side of your body. If it's too much for you, you can rest your arm along your body.

After holding for 3 or 5 breaths, repeat on the other side.

NAVASANA (BOAT POSE)

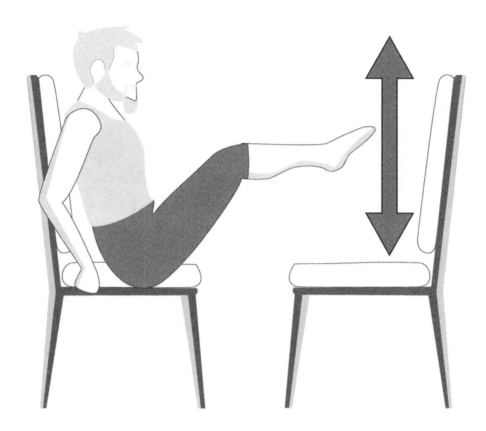

It is a balancing pose that strengthens the abdominal muscles, back and hip flexors, while toning the digestive organs. It also gives strength and flexibility to your legs and hip joints.

Start by sitting in the mat chair with your knees facing forward and your feet flat on the floor.
Move to the edge of the chair; lean back slightly, and place your hands behind you on the chair. As you exhale, lift your feet off the floor and bring your knees towards your chest. During the entire process, keep your back straight and engage your abdominal muscle. If you find this posture difficult, use another chair to support.

Continue to breathe deeply while holding this position for 30 seconds to one minute. To release, slowly lower your feet to the floor and sit straight.

Repeat two or three times, never forgetting to breathe deeply!

HIGH ALTAR

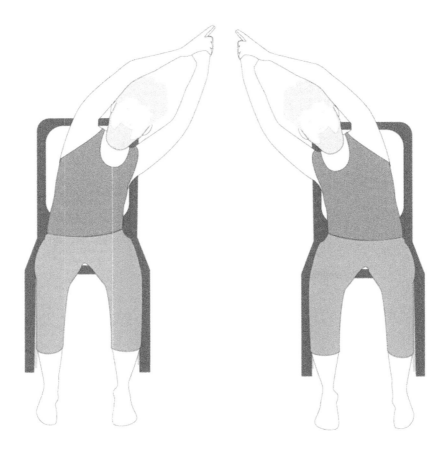

This pose helps to stretch the spine, stretch the back muscles and energize the body.

Start by sitting high at the end of the chair.

On each inhalation, raise your hands over your head and reach as high above your head as possible. Also, stretch across the spine as far as possible.

When you have reached the stretch position, inhale, contract your abdominal muscles and bend your torso to the right without losing the stretch or rotating your spine. Hold for 3-4 breaths.

Slowly, return to the center and repeat towards the left side.

SPINAL TWISTS

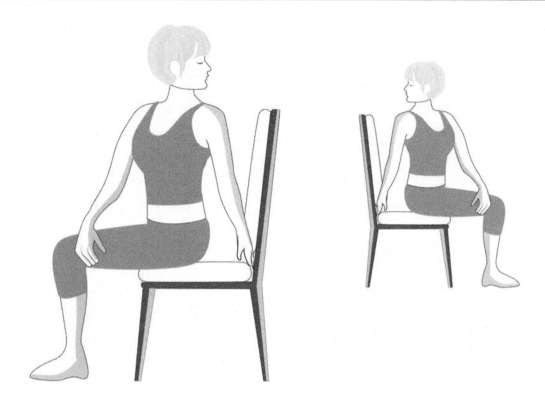

Start by sitting comfortably in the chair, placing your feet on the ground.
Then start taking a deep inhalation.

As you exhale, gently rotate your torso to the right, turning your head as well. Place your left hand on your right knee and your right hand on the back of the chair.

Hold this twist for 3-4 breaths. Then gently return to the neutral position.

At this point, do this very same twist on the left side. Gently rotate your torso and head to the left, placing your right hand on your left knee and your left hand on the back of the chair. Inhale and exhale during the process.

Hold this position for 3-4 breaths. Then return to the starting position; proceed to alternate the two rotations for at least 2-3 minutes.

VIRABHADRASANA I (WARRIOR POSE)

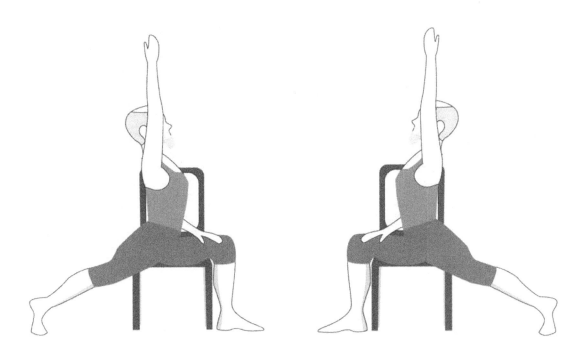

Virabhadra was a warrior hero born from the hair of the god Shiva to take revenge for the offense suffered by Daksa, the father of his wife. He is usually depicted in front of the temples as a guardian.

That is why the word literally means 'position of the stationary hero or grandiose hero': because it acts as a guardian of our health. Among the benefits of this pose, in fact, we can find a strengthening of the ankles, legs, shoulders, and back, but also a greater focus and concentration on body, mind, and even soul. Additionally, this pose helps strengthen your balance, helping you avoid falls.

Sit towards the left side of the chair and open your right leg at a 90-degree angle to the front of the chair. Open your left leg and reach behind you, keeping only a slight bend in the knee. Open the trunk on the right.

Press the toes of the left foot to the floor, heel up. Press firmly on both feet and try to lift the weight off the chair. If the pose is comfortable, raise your hands and hold here.

Repeat on both sides.

WARRIOR II

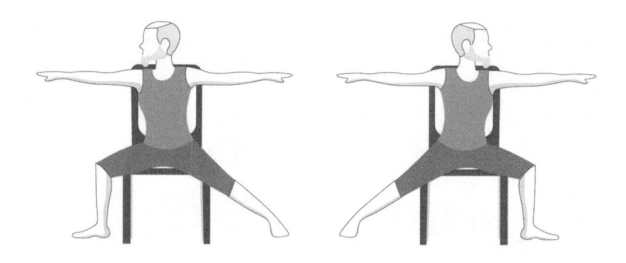

Just like Warrior I, Warrior II can also be modified for a chair.

Sit towards the left side of the chair and open your right leg at a 90-degree angle to the front of the chair.

Open your left leg and reach for it to the left, keeping only a slight bend in the knee. Keep your chest open forward.

Press firmly on both feet and try to lift the weight off the chair. If the pose is comfortable, bring your hands together and stretch your arms to opposite sides of the room.

Repeat on both sides.

WARRIOR III

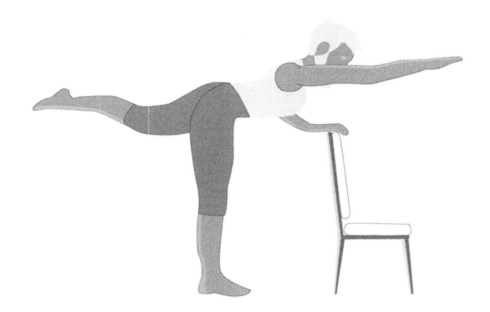

Position yourself about 1 meter from the back of the chair (with the seat on the opposite side to which you are).

As you exhale, tilt your chest forward, placing your weight on your front leg and arms, which are supported by the chair.
At this point, slowly extend the opposite leg off the ground.
Lift your leg even more by keeping it parallel to the floor
Stabilize yourself on the supporting leg while keeping the knee slightly bent if necessary, but without overextending the back, which must remain aligned with the rear leg.
When you feel stable, try to remove the arm opposite the stretched leg from the chair, placing it at the same height.
For balance, help yourself by fixing a point in front of you.
Hold the position until one feels secure and firm.

To exit the position, exhale by raising your arms above your head and placing one foot next to the other in Tadasana.
Repeat on the other side, trying to stay at the same time.

It is normal that the two sides do not behave in the same way, and there is an easier one. Smile and try again!

VIPARITA VIRABHADRASANA II (REVERSE WARRIOR II POSE)

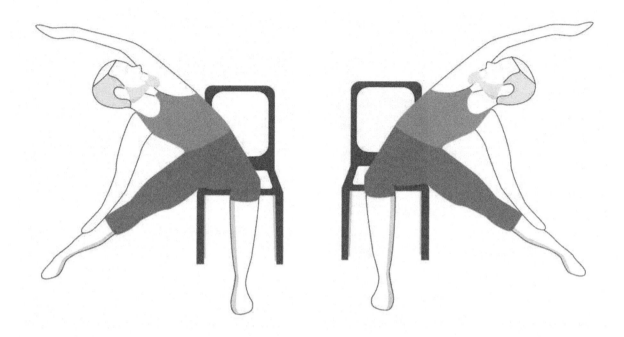

Assume the position of Warrior II: try to flex the knee well and extend the leg behind as much as possible by contracting the quadriceps.

Then root your feet on the ground, soften your shoulders and imagine that you want to touch something by stretching both arms in opposite directions.

The abdomen is well contracted, and the spine elongated.

Keeping the legs still and being careful not to extend the flexed knee, bring the hand to the extended leg and let the other arm go over your head.

You will feel the chest open and stretch.

If you don't have issues with your neck, look up and increase the breadth of your breath.

ARDHA KAPOTASANA (SEATED PIGEON POSE)

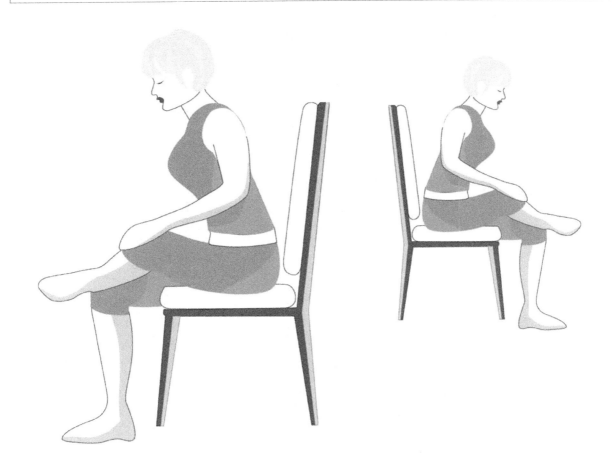

This classic pose is great for opening your hips. Using a chair as a support can make it much more accessible for people with narrow hips.

Sit towards the left side of the chair and open your right leg at a 90-degree angle to the front of the chair.

Rotate your chest to the right at a 45-degree angle from the front of the chair.

Bring your right leg into the chair, closing the joint in half.

Reach your left leg back and press your toes to the floor, heel up.

N.B. *Careful for people with knee pain or very stiff hips.*

GARUDASANA (EAGLE POSE)

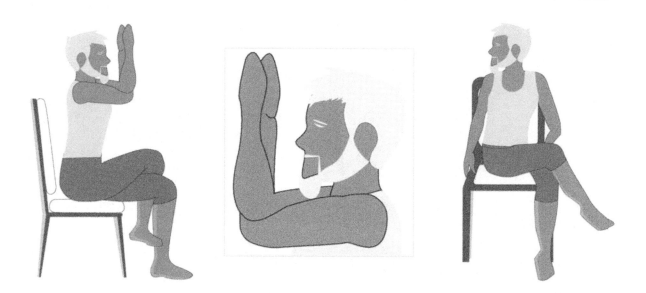

This is a great variation of a classic yoga pose that can be performed on a chair. When done regularly, it is a great way to relieve sciatic pain. This pose also helps to open your upper back, shoulders, elbows, and wrists.

Sit with your feet hip-distance apart, firmly on the floor. Remember to always keep your back straight.

Cross your left leg over your right leg so that the knees are close together. If mobility allows, move your right foot slightly forward and wrap your left toes around your left leg. Take your arms out at shoulder height.

Cross your left elbow over your right elbow and keep your arms at an angle of 90 degrees, with your fingers pointing towards the ceiling. Bend your elbows and bring your palms together.

Lift your elbows as you spread your shoulders. Inhale as you do this and hold the position for at least five seconds. Exhale and release, repeating in the other direction.

If you cannot touch your palms, do a modified version: press the back of your hands instead. Lift your elbows towards the ceiling and make sure to relax your shoulders and the face muscles.

Chapter 10
Easy Chair Yoga Routines for Seniors

Senior Restorative Flow - Beginner

Who: for you, if you want to start your day with energy and intention.
What: your chair.
When: in the morning to start the day; in the afternoon; before bed.
Where: at home.
How: gently, without forcing the movements.
Why: set your intention for the practice: 'Today I choose this because …'

Hold each pose for 5 deep breaths.

1. Anjali Mudra (Pg. 32)
2. Shoulder Releases (Pg. 24)
3. Neck Releases (Pg. 23)
4. Side bends - Right Side (Pg. 37)
5. Side bends - Left Side (Pg. 37)
6. Twist - Right Side (Pg. 51)
7. Twist - Left Side (Pg. 51)
8. Cobra Pose (Pg. 46)
9. Raised Hands (Pg. 33)
10. Forward Fold (Pg. 35)
11. Pigeon Pose - Right Side (Pg. 56)
12. Pigeon Pose - Left Side (Pg. 56)
13. Savasana (Pg. 43-45)

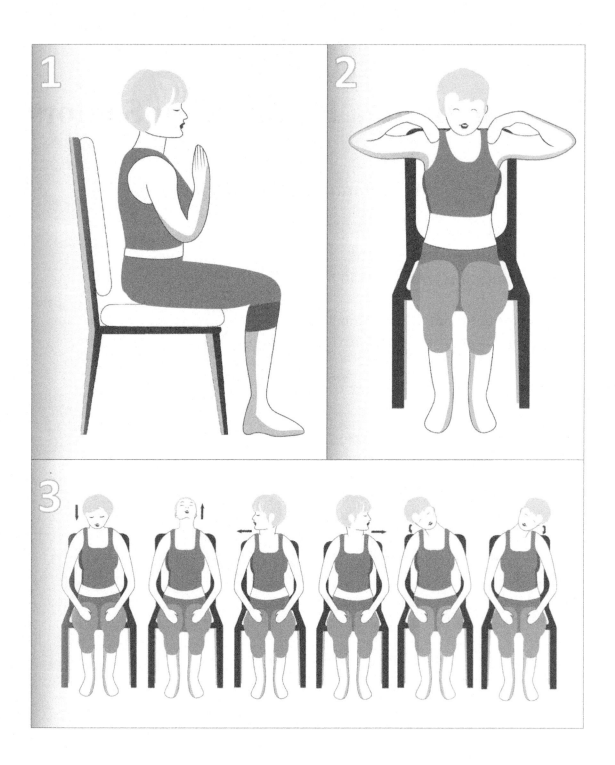

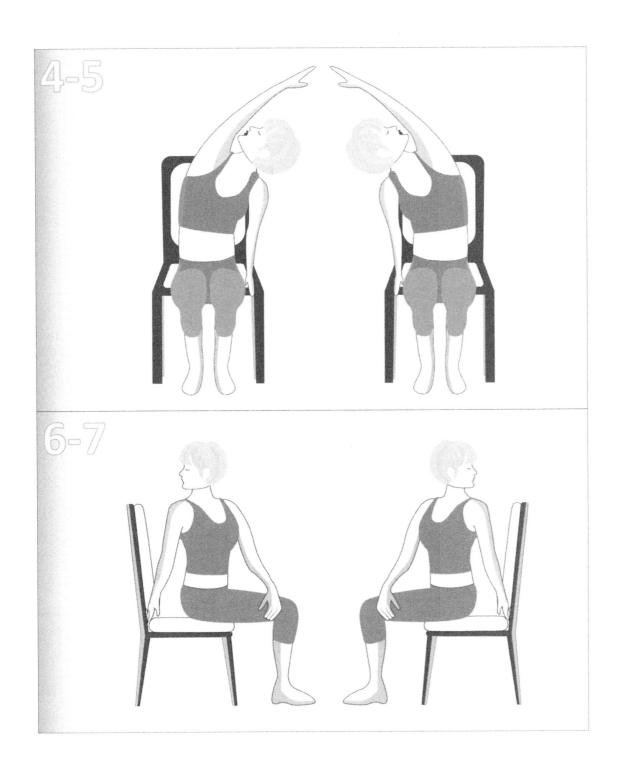

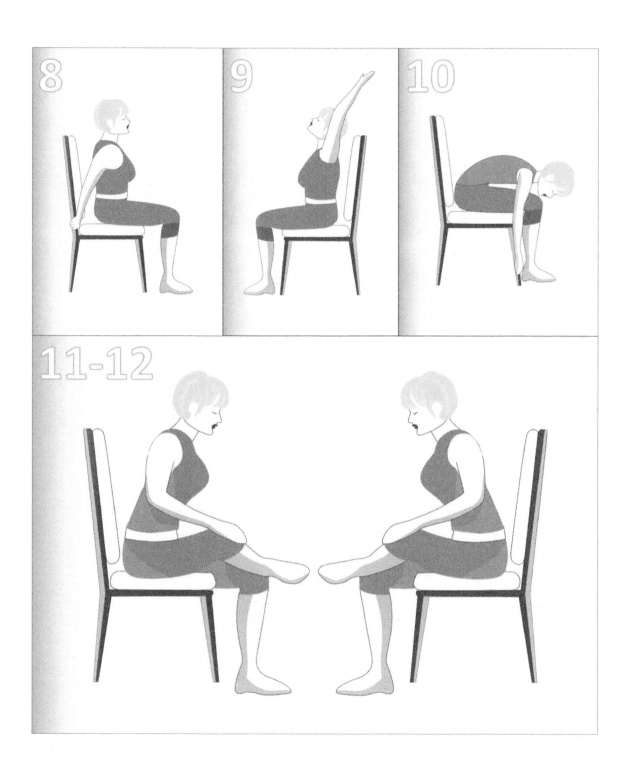

61

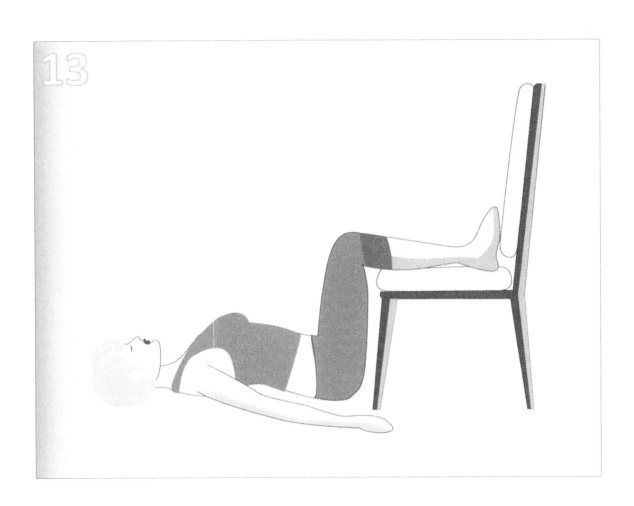

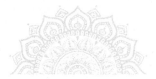

Surya Namaskar (Sun Salutation Flow) - Intermediate

Who: for you, if you want to start your day with energy and intention.
What: your chair.
When: in the morning to start the day; in the afternoon.
Where: at home.
How: gently, without forcing the movements.
Why: set your intention for the practice: 'Today I choose this because …'

Hold each pose for 5 deep breaths.

1.   Anjali Mudra (Pg. 32)
2.   Raised Hands (Pg. 33)
3.   Forward Fold (Pg. 35-36)
4.   Knee to Chest - Right Side (Pg. 34)
5.   Ragdoll on the Chair - Right Side (Pg. 35-36)
6.   Raised Hands (Pg. 33)
7.   Forward Fold (Pg. 35-36)
8.   Knee to Chest - Left Side (Pg. 34)
9.   Ragdoll on the Chair - Left Side (Pg. 35-36)
10. Raised Hands (Pg. 33)
11. Forward Fold (Pg. 35-36)
12. Raised Hands (Pg. 33)
13. Anjali Mudra (Pg. 32)
14. Savasana (Pg. 43-45)

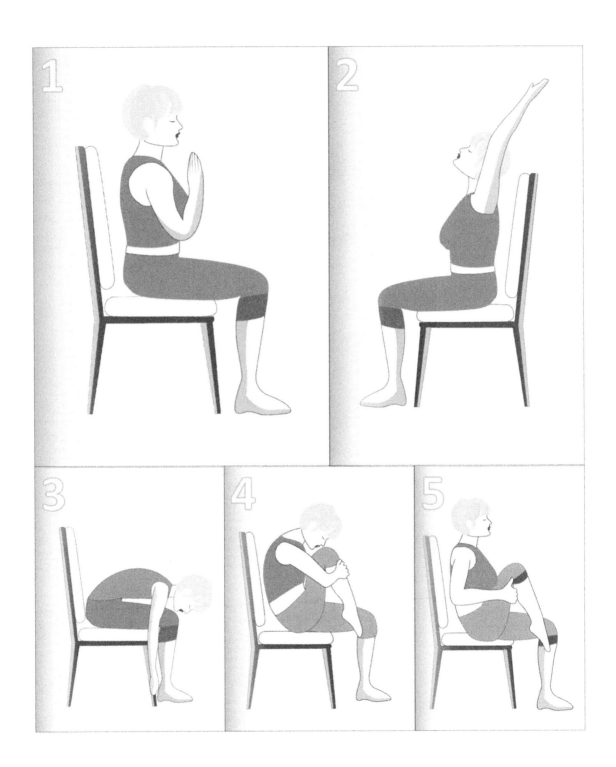

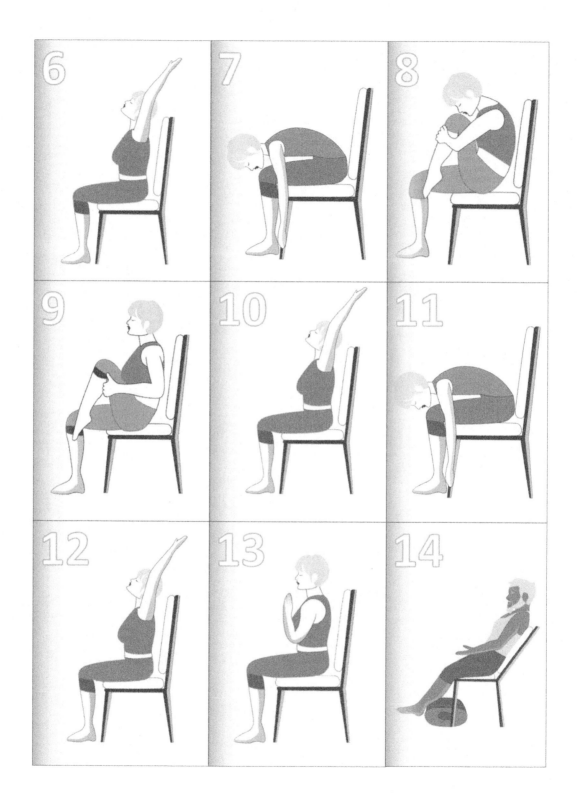

Moon salutation flow - Intermediate

Who: for you, if you want to end your day with inspiration and gratitude.
What: your chair.
When: in the afternoon; before bed.
Where: at home.
How: gently, without forcing the movements.
Why: set your intention for the practice: 'Today I choose this because …'

Hold each pose for 5 deep breaths.

1.   Anjali Mudra (Pg. 32)
2.   Raised Hands (Pg. 33)
3.   Goddess Pose (Pg. 39)
4.   Extended Side Angle - Right Side (Pg. 48)
5.   Warrior I - Right Side (Pg. 52)
6.   Reverse Warrior II - Right Side (Pg. 55)
7.   Warrior I - Left Side (Pg. 52)
8.   Reverse Warrior II - Left Side (Pg. 55)
9.   Extended Side Angle - Left Side (Pg. 48)
10.   Goddess Pose (Pg. 39)
11.   Anjali Mudra (Pg. 32)
12.   Savasana (Pg. 43-45)

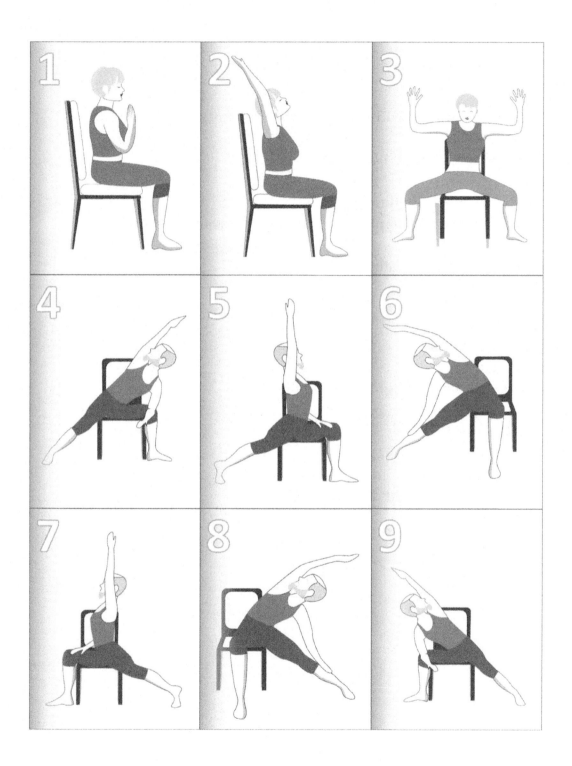

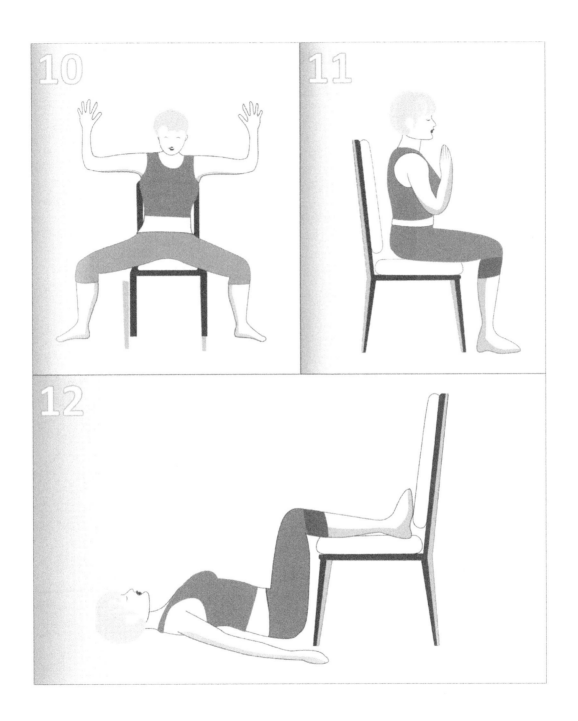

BOOK 2:
STRETCHING EXERCISES FOR SENIORS

Chapter 1
Flexibility is The Key

Stretching workout is considered one of the most effective strategies for the well-being of elderly people, which is why it is often also practiced as a daily workout. In fact, it is a physical activity suitable for the elderly but also for all those people who practice sports occasionally or professionally.

Gentle gymnastics involves slow and gradual movements that allow you to train the body without excessively stressing muscles and joints.

Most seniors are not trained and do not play sports; therefore, doing intense exercises can cause pain and discomfort or, in some cases, even damage to the musculoskeletal system.

With gentle gymnastics, on the other hand, it is possible to train without the risk of getting hurt, allowing anyone, even those with difficulty moving or walking, not to give up physical activity.

In the course of the Chapters, we will see just some simple but fundamental stretching exercises and what are the benefits of each of these in your life.

But first: why is stretching so important for everyone, especially for seniors?

Elderly people are subject to a greater risk of diseases related to the wear and tear of the joints and muscles. That's why stretching for seniors is a great way to prevent these health problems.

Stretching is certainly very useful at any age. If this practice is included in your daily routine, the subject will, without a doubt, have a better functionality of his own body.

When the body carries out very little physical activity, the joints tend to stiffen, muscle weakness increases, and blood flow is reduced.

In this sense, from being a simple sequence of exercises, stretching becomes a necessary need of the body to feel good and be able to perform its motor functions, regain flexibility.

Let's start by clarifying the real concept of the word flexibility.

Flexibility is the condition enjoyed when muscles and joints are mobile and elastic.

The joints move thanks to the strength of the muscles, but over time these lose elasticity, and the movements become more difficult. Stretching practiced regularly helps to delay and slow down this process.

For example, someone who has worked at a desk for years with poor posture will likely suffer from stiff back and legs. The famous 'desk' posture causes the hip flexors (the anterior muscles that join the thigh to the pelvis) to shorten and the back muscles to stretch, causing the spine to curve forward.

Likewise, as the years go by, it is normal for mobility to decrease. This is a problem because this skill is essential for having an active and quality life: it allows you to get up, move and do whatever you want (and without pain). Fortunately, mobility is a function that can be worked on: the loss of mobility has more to do with the change in lifestyles that tend to take over at a certain point in life rather than with the change of body. Therefore, you can avoid many risks and harmful consequences if you work hard to stay active and mobile.

The best way to improve flexibility is to practice gentle, regular stretching that gradually increases joint mobility. So the ideal is to practice gentle stretching every day; 10 minutes of exercise are enough to maintain good flexibility and prevent future problems.

Furthermore, it should be remembered that if you practice regular physical activity at the end of each training session, general stretching should be practiced because precisely by working, the muscles contract and shorten, and the body loses flexibility.

Stretching when the muscles are still 'warm' and more reactive reduces the shortening phenomenon, can help disperse the lactic acid that accumulates under exertion, and reduces the risk of contracting injuries.

Chapter 2
Mobility: Your Asset for Healthy Aging

Mobility refers to how well the joints move through their full range of motion; more simply, it indicates how a person moves, for example, how much and how he can extend and flex an elbow or ankle. The more mobile you are, the more you can move and walk freely and easily. This is essential for staying healthy and living independently, without anyone's help, according to the National Institute on Aging (NIA).

People with good mobility, for example, can raise their arms to reach the closet, go up and down stairs (which indicates good ankle mobility), and bend over to pick something up from the floor (a sign of good hips, knees, and ankle mobility).

Lack of mobility results in less autonomy and independence and a greater risk of falls, illness, loss of function, and even death. The individual may feel stiff and sore without good joint mobility, and performing daily activities or playing sports becomes more difficult. Losing mobility can be a major drag on quality of life. Fortunately, it is possible to improve mobility and range of motion, reducing pain, anxiety, and depression and improving the ability to perform daily activities and personal care routines.

Some loss of mobility is normal with the passage of age: in fact, a natural consequence of aging is the breakdown of collagen, the structure that holds water, which provides fluid and elasticity to the joints. This loss makes it harder for the joints to access their full range of motion.

In addition, certain conditions become more common with age, such as hypertension, heart disease, heart failure, diabetes, rheumatoid arthritis, and osteoarthritis, which are associated with a loss of mobility. Age-related sarcopenia and muscle loss can also contribute to decreased mobility.

However, the main reason why joint mobility decreases with age is represented by incorrect habits: a sedentary lifestyle and repetitive movements in first place. For example, continuous typing on a keyboard shortens the muscles in the front of the chest; if you are also leaning forward (a common posture at a desk), your back muscles will stretch excessively.

Over the years, if nothing is done to counteract that habitual activity, the muscles on one side of one joint will chronically shorten, and the muscles on the other side will chronically stretch. The danger is that this can cause wear and tear on the joints, which, in the long term, can lead to chronic pain. Also, if you are not physically active, your joints are not stimulated to move through their full range of motion.

How to preserve and improve mobility with age? A person is not condemned to frailty and immobility just because they get older if they are willing to stay active and prioritize wellbeing. Staying active and living a healthy lifestyle is one of the best things you can do for the present and the future. To improve mobility, you can also try some challenges or simple daily routines (we will address this topic later). Here are the best strategies to be adopted to train mobility.

Stay active

Do what you can to have an active lifestyle. If you move, you can compensate for some of the loss of mobility due to aging. And that doesn't mean training for running the marathon or doing high-intensity interval training (although you can).

In a study published in 2021, seniors who did light-intensity daily physical activity (gardening, walking, or even drying dishes) were up to 40% less likely to develop mobility problems over six years than those who were less active.

Pro tip: one of the simplest and best exercises is walking - this is a great place to start. The person should plan daily walks, starting with short sessions, up to 30 minutes daily. On busy days, do what you can. Every step counts.

Diversify your workouts

Finding a workout you love is great, but doing the same daily exercises isn't ideal for joint mobility. It is recommended to engage in different training sessions on different days of the week: a combination of different activities such as walking, strength training, chair yoga, or core workouts will move the joints in all possible ways.

For example, if you only train with your bicycle, your joints will move into one position, and that can cause your hips, back, and chest to become tense and sore. You can reduce this risk by opening the front of the body through strength and yoga.

Don't always sit down

Those who spend long periods of time in a sitting position for professional or personal reasons must move often. For example, they can stand up and/or walk five minutes every hour. The earlier you start this habit, the better, but it's never too late.

Moreover, standing up to interrupt time spent sitting engages the large skeletal muscles and triggers thousands of muscle contractions if repeated consistently throughout the day.

Stretching, of course

Stretching that involves the shoulders, spine, hips, and calves can combat chronic stiffness that contributes to loss of mobility in the elderly. Stretching with static (bend and hold) and dynamic (fluid) stretches a great opportunity to move joints in optimal ways.

Be careful not to push too hard in the stretches so as not to damage the joints. The goal is to feel a slight and pleasant stretch of the muscles.

Chapter 3
6 Benefits of Gentle Stretching

Stretching for seniors can be especially helpful. Practicing it correctly allows you to reduce muscle tension and make movements more fluid, improve flexibility, and acquire greater balance.

It is also ideal for those who tend to suffer from muscle tears: thanks to its relaxing action on the muscles, stretching allows the elderly to move better, removing the risk of muscle accidents.

It is also possible to do gentle gymnastics for the elderly to lose weight, with an exercise program aimed at weight loss, without making people in old age run the risk of suffering trauma and injuries. The important thing, however, is that it is practiced correctly, respecting the limits of each person.

Let's look at some of the benefits of this type of gymnastics and why it is the best seniors' health strategy.

1 - Stretching helps prevent disease
Medical science tells us that prevention is essential at all stages of life and, in particular, in old age. Many studies have shown that the elderly who exercise reduce the risk of getting sick or contracting typical age-related diseases.

Gentle gymnastics becomes a valuable prevention tool, helping the body protect itself from specific diseases such as osteoarthritis, a progressive and degenerative disease of the joints - cartilage and surrounding tissues - frequent in the adult population. 10% suffer from it, of which 50% are over 50. In particular, it occurs twice as often in women, with a higher incidence of overweight or obese people.

2 - Stretching helps slow down the aging process
Aging is a progressive physiological process that alters cells and tissues, with aesthetic and functional consequences.

The muscles, in old age, reduce the tone, and it is thanks to gentle gymnastics that it is possible to counteract this phenomenon. Exercising preserves the ability to walk independently, as the muscle is always active and in motion.

3 - Stretching promotes joint well-being
Joints also tend to undergo functional changes, and many older adults have difficulty making larger movements. With gentle gymnastics exercises, it is possible to keep the joints in training, performing slow and gradual movements that do not overstimulate the joints, thus avoiding inflammation and pain.

4 - Stretching improves mood
Gentle gymnastics also offers psychological benefits. It is known that physical activity improves mood and greatly reduces the risk of depression or the appearance of other psychological disorders.

5 - Stretching improves balance
By constantly performing the exercises, it is possible to observe an improvement in balance in the elderly and/or a reduction in problems related to aging. Many accidental falls are due to poor balance, and gentle gymnastics for the elderly can be useful to reduce the risk of domestic accidents.

6 - Stretching means well-being at 360°
Daily stretching and an active lifestyle positively affect the health of the elderly. Both physically and mentally. Motor activity increases the body's functions at 360 °, improving the system:
• skeletal muscle;
• respiratory;
• urinary;
• cardio-circulatory.

As well as, no less important, cognitive and psychic functions in general. The result is a refinement of intellectual performance, the alleviation of anxiety symptoms, and improved sleep and mood.

Chapter 4
Stretching for Seniors: How to Start

Warming up is essential

To be carried out correctly, every stretching session for the elderly must be preceded by an adequate period of warming up the body.

5-10 minutes of slow walking is often enough to prepare the body and muscles for physical activity. Warming up, in fact, allows you to activate the muscles in order to prepare them for subsequent physical activity, reducing the risk of muscle tears.

A correct practice

At the end of the warm-up, you can start doing the proper stretching exercises. These can be aimed at stretching the back and leg muscles, for example, loosening the shoulders, maintaining balance, and so on.

The important thing is to perform them slowly, without sudden movements, avoiding exercises aimed at stressing muscles or parts of the body where the pain is felt. It is equally important that the muscle stretching lasts for a minimum of 15-20 seconds and that during the exercise you breathe normally.

By relying on practicing a few simple exercises, you can improve the balance and fluidity of movements: stretching can be a great way to keep fit, flexible, and happy in the process!

To set up a specific motor path, you may need a specialist assessment that involves various professionals: the orthopedist, the geriatrician, the physiotherapist, the osteopath, as well as the neurologist, and the psychologist.

Gentle gymnastics aims to maintain motor skills, reactivate the muscles, and release some diseases affecting the joints, neck, etc. The ultimate goal is to preserve and, if possible, improve daily autonomy and self-care.

Stretching activity includes free body exercises with the aid of special tools, breathing, relaxation, and easy muscle activities.

In this sense, it is the set of movements designed to extend the upper and lower limbs, the spine, and the trunk.

However, the following exercises can be performed at home in complete tranquility. That's why you are here!

Follow the simple instructions for each exercise or during the various workouts, move slowly and at your own pace, especially if you are just starting, and ... follow your flow of flexibility!

What you need to start

Before starting your workout, prepare yourself well and make sure you have the tools for your workout:
• comfortable, breathable, and stretchy clothes;
• a pair of chairs with a comfortable back and seat (we will see how to use them later);
• a semi-rigid ball;
• a belt with a noose or rubber stretch bands;
• two towels, one for sweat and one for the chair;
• your best smile!

Best Tips before stretching out

Senior people need to take some precautions before starting to stretch to avoid injury or possible injury. Pay close attention to the following recommendations:
• Do not strain your body too much. If for some reason you cannot perform the exercise in its entirety, do not force yourself;
• Get as far as you can; with practice, you will improve. You shouldn't feel pain when you stretch, maybe a little tension, but never pain;
• Relax your muscles: during stretching exercises, the muscles must be relaxed and not tense. In this way, they can stretch and oxygenate without problems;
• Perform the exercises correctly. You must try to have a technique that allows you to perform the exercises in the correct way possible.

It is very vital to remember that, like any exercise, there is always a risk of injury. Consult your doctor, especially before starting any exercise program, bearing in mind your age and health situation, to find out which exercises are best for you.

That becomes crucial for those with walking difficulties or relapsing from surgery.

Chapter 5
Types of Stretching

When we sleep, our muscles relax, the blood flow decreases, our whole body temperature drops, and the heart rate slows down. So morning stretching is important to wake up our body. Furthermore, if we are lying in the same position all night, the muscles tend to contract.

So stretching in the morning is essential to wake up our body because we, like any living being, instinctively tend to try it as soon as we wake up.

Let's go immediately to find out why stretching in the morning is essential, starting from the advantages you will see on the first day. Before accompanying you in the exercises, we want to give you five simple rules to do the best stretching and provide you unstoppable charge during the morning.

1. While relaxing the affected part, breathe deeply, inhaling with your nose and exhaling with your mouth, and try to lengthen the exhalation phase. You will feel that the whole body will be more relaxed, and the muscles will relax more easily;

2. As soon as you wake up, your body temperature is low, and the muscle bands tend to contract, so try to be cautious and don't continue to stretch a muscle chain if it starts to hurt;

3. Do not exceed 20-30 seconds of stretch per position;

4. Physiologically, we are asymmetrical; the right side of our body is slightly different than the left, so the muscles will also have other contractures, so perform an asymmetrical stretch focusing more on the contracted parts;

5. Use comfortable clothing that allows for wide-ranging movements without blocking deep breathing.

Here are the best stretching exercises and routines for your flexibility and happiness!

RISE AND SHINE MORNING STRETCHING (5 MINUTES)

When we sleep, our muscles relax, the blood flow decreases, our whole body temperature drops, and the heart rate slows down. So morning stretching is important to wake up our body. Furthermore, if we are lying in the same position all night, the muscles tend to contract.

So stretching in the morning is essential to wake up our body because we, like any living being, instinctively tend to try it as soon as we wake up.

Let's go immediately to find out why stretching in the morning is essential, starting from the advantages you will see on the first day. Before accompanying you in the exercises, we want to give you five simple rules to do the best stretching and provide you unstoppable charge during the morning.

1. CHEST OUT / BELLY IN

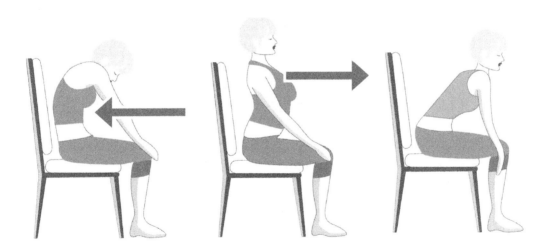

Sit on the chair with both feet flat on the floor. Sit close to the edge of the chair.
Put your hands on your knees or on the top of your thighs. Breathe in.

During an inhalation, slowly arch your back, bringing your chest forward and pulling your tailbone and shoulders back. Then arch the spine by pushing the chest out and as you exhale forcefully, bring the shoulders back to their place and continue like this.
Inhale and exhale as you arch your torso downwards. Repeat 3 to 5 times.

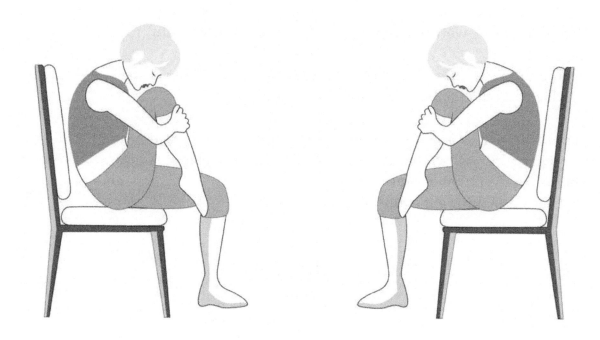

Sit on the chair: your knees are bent, and your feet are flat on the floor.

Gently raise one bent knee up enough so you can grasp your lower leg with both hands. Interlace your fingers just under the knee. If you're doing the two-legged version, bring one leg up and then the other.

Gently pull your bent knee or knees toward your trunk using your hands. Hold for a few seconds.

Return your leg to the floor. If you are doing it with one leg at a time, repeat on the other side.

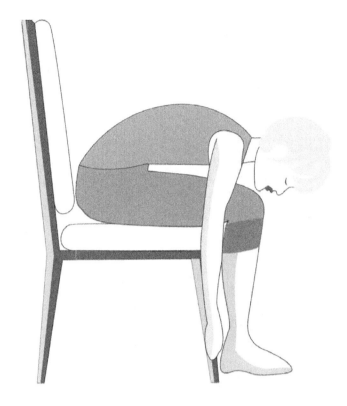

Inhale and raise your arms.

As you exhale, lean forward, resting your torso on your thighs.

If possible, place your hands on the floor and dangle your head. Rest in this position for a few breaths.

To exit, straighten your arms in front of you above your head and come up.

Repeat three times in total, and the last time you bend forward, stay there.

4. LIKE A BUTTERFLY

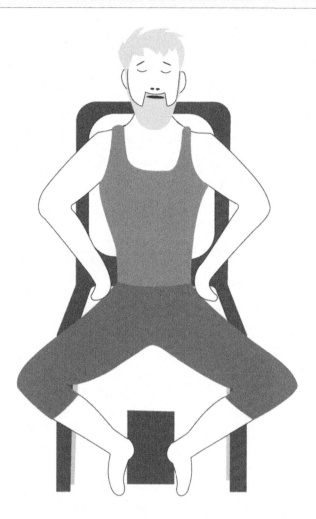

Take your yoga blocks before sitting down. Then place them in the highest, vertical length and place your feet on top slowly.

The soles of the feet touch, while the knees fall sideways.

Don't force the opening: let gravity help you!

Bring your hands clasped to your hips, maintaining the position, and inhale and exhale for 3-5 breaths.

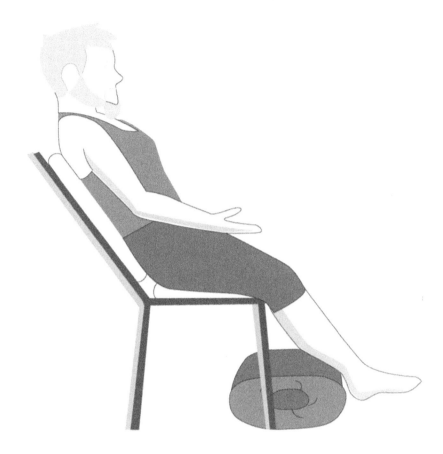

Sit on the chair with your back flat and your pelvis slightly forward.

Extend your legs forward, almost as an extension of the rest of your body, with your feet relaxed and your heels touching the ground.

Bring your hands to your belly, with your shoulders completely relaxed. Relax the muscles of the neck, face, and mouth. Breathe naturally.

Now close your eyes and bring your attention to your breath. Focus on filling your lungs evenly, right and left for a few minutes. Consciously expand the chest upwards and outwards as you inhale; release your breath.

Breath slowly. The practice of conscious breathing, through support, will have a calming effect on the nervous system.

Still in Bed Morning Stretching (5 minutes)

1. WARM-UP

Before doing any stretching movements, it is good to warm up the area of your pelvic muscles and ligaments.

To do so, there are several way: you can use a heating pad or a rubber hot water bottle or your hands.

Gently place them on your stomach and breathe naturally. The heat will be the first signal you give your body to tell it it's time to get going.

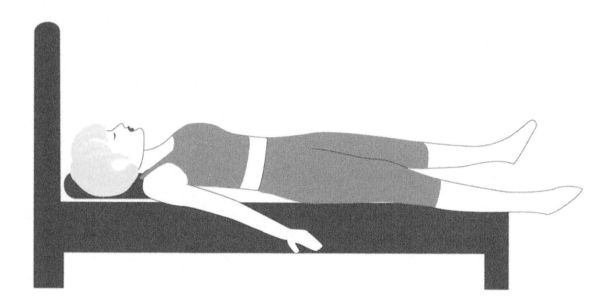

2. KNEE EXTENSION

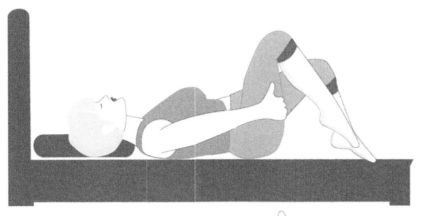

Lie on your back, removing the pillow from under your head if it is more appropriate for you.

Bring one knee towards your chest and keep the opposite leg stretched out on the bed.

Grasp the lower leg and squeeze it towards the chest.

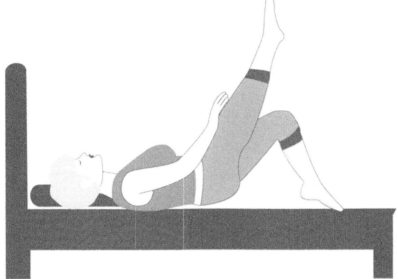

Hold the position for a variable time between 10 and 30 seconds, depending on your level of training and the feeling of comfort experienced. Next, lift the leg at the top. It does not need to be completely extended or remain in a painful position: see how far you can go, dedicate 4-5 breaths to this movement and then come back with the leg bent and stretched out on the bed.

Return to the original position and repeat with the other leg. Do 2 to 4 repetitions on each side.

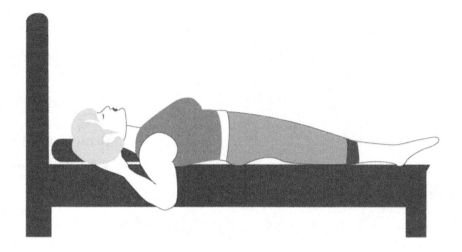

Lie in bed, with your back fully adhering to the sheets. At this point, extend your legs and let your feet touch each other, with the toes pointing towards the opposite wall (the dancer's feet, basically).

Maintaining this position and with your shoulders and neck muscles relaxed, move the tips of your feet back and forth for 30 seconds.

When finished, move your ankles freely to awaken the joint.

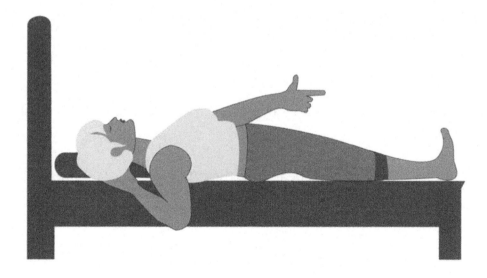

4. HIP LUBRIFICATION

Lie in bed, with your back fully adhering to the sheets. At this point, bends the knees while keeping your feet on the bed.

Keeping your back attached to the blankets, bring your knees to the left first and turn your head to look at the right shoulder.

Hold for 15 seconds, then do the same on the opposite side. This position is one of the best stretching exercises for the neck!

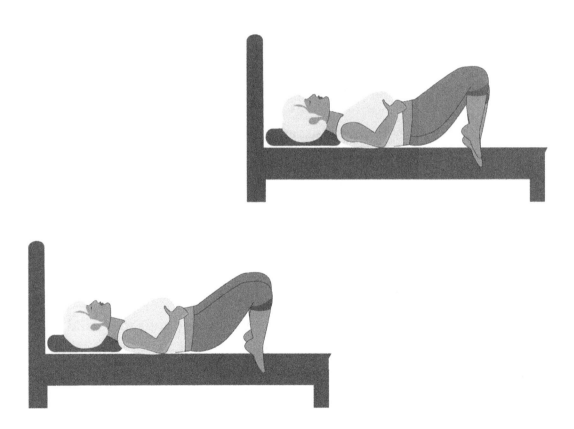

5. GLUTES EXTENSIONS

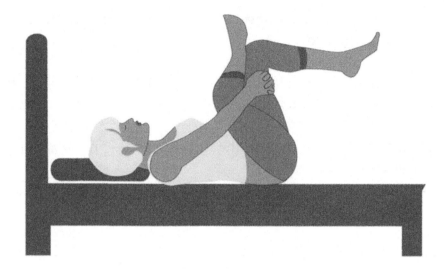

Lie on your back: arms at your sides and palms facing down.

Cross one ankle over the other knee. Raise one leg, then cross it over the other, keeping your knee bent. Rest your ankle on your thigh, just above the opposite knee, with your knee at almost a right angle.

Feel your lower back and make sure you're still lying flat on the bed. You don't want to arch your lower back.

Clasp your hands across your thighs. Grasp the lower leg just below the knee by running one hand across the raised leg and the other by your side.
Embrace your knee with your hands and gently push to lift your knee and foot off the floor. Pull your body in as far as you can comfortably and feel the stretch.

If you push the inner thigh of the raised leg with your elbow, you can also open the hips.
Make sure you have all four corners of your torso pressed onto the bed.
Stay here for 30 -45 seconds. Then repeat everything on the other side.

6. BRIDGE

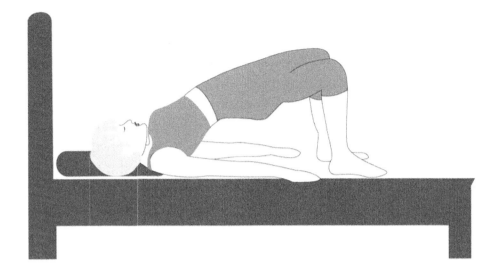

Lie on your back: your arms at your sides and palms facing down. Then bend your knees, rests your feet on the floor below the knees, and spread your legs to the same width as the hips.

Press your feet to the floor, lift your hips and create a straight line from the knees to the shoulders. Then squeeze the glute and pulls the navel back towards the spine.

Bring the weight of the body on the shoulder blades and the upper back, do not keep the load of the body resting on the neck.

You can perform the basic bridge statically by holding the position for 20 to 30 seconds, or actively bringing your hips up and down without touching the floor, 15-30 times.

Repeat the exercise for 2-3 laps. You can also perform the basic bridge while resting on your toes or heels.

Now that you are done close your eyes and lie down for a few moments, thanking your body for what it has done. Keep your eyes closed, sit still for a few moments and then proceed with your day!

WARM UP: STANDING POSES BEFORE EXERCISES

Gentle Stretching is always designed to favor the body and not overload it. Therefore all those practices that bring pain are not recommended. Exercises are not challenges to your possibilities; doing physical activity does not mean suffering to obtain results at any cost, and excessive effort is neither a means to obtain physical beauty nor to punish yourself for not having done physical activity first - perhaps for several years or for a lifetime.

Before looking at some useful and targeted exercises, let's focus on this last point.

The body must always be listened to. If you feel muscle resistance or pain, stop and rest. Physical activity for the elderly must be the slow but constant search for well-being, vitality, and opportunity. Not a way to save yourself from disease.

Performing the exercises with good company can be an excellent deterrent to regaining vitality, sharing mutual efforts, and finding support in other people.

Physical movement, therefore, has multiple benefits on the individual, being a social aggregator and an enhancer of the functionality of muscles, joints, and bones. From the first weeks, it will have a beneficial effect on the body, and this will positively affect the mind of the elderly. Soon many manage to tie their shoes and put on their socks by themselves, take a glass from a high shelf or take their grandchild for a walk without getting too tired.

It is a false cliché that 'the older you get, the less you have to move'. Instead, moving the right personalized paths proportional to the specific case is necessary. They can then, over time, be adjusted to progress more and more.

Here then, this group of standing exercises will be useful when you want to warm up to move, train, or even try your hand at normal household chores such as gardening, painting, or a bike ride.

Equipment you will need:

• your goodwill :);

• stairs or steps;

• a wall;

• a mat;

• a chair;

• light weights for the ankles.

1. WALL SQUATS

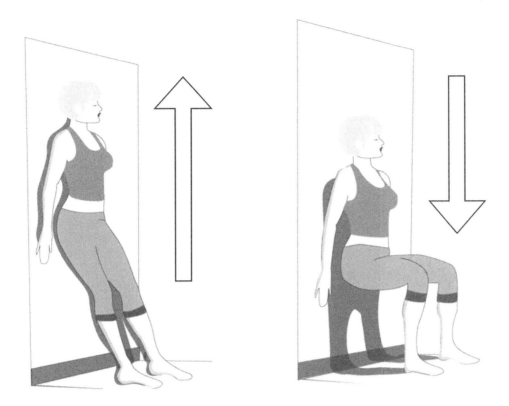

Lean your back against a wall. Take two steps forward.

Spread your legs slightly apart and move your feet about 60cm away from the wall. The feet should be approximately 15 cm apart.

Slide your back down against the wall.

Bend your knees 90 degrees, so your thighs are parallel to the floor. You will have to look like you are sitting in an invisible chair. The knees must be aligned with the ankles; check that they do not lean forward. If necessary, move your back higher or lower to position them correctly. Straighten your legs and come back to your feet, letting your back slide against the wall. Rest for 30 seconds.

Aim to repeat this five times and hold the squat position for 20 seconds each time. If your muscles are too tired to allow you to continue, stop the exercise and move forward.

2. HIP ABDUCTION

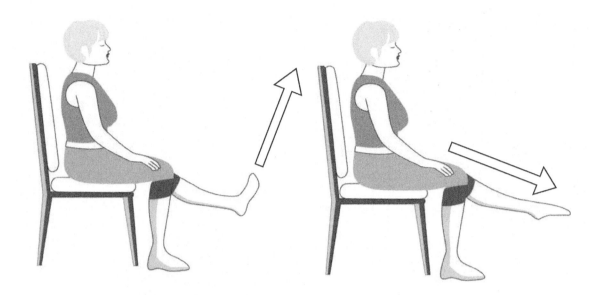

Stand up with your hand on the chair, wearing your **ankle weights.**
Keep a stand firm position and the foot touching.

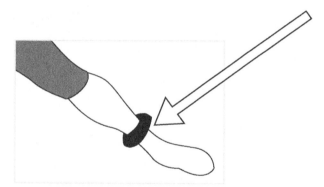

At this point, inhale and put your belly in a while extending your leg out. Try to maintain the hips pointing straight in front of you while raising your leg up on the side.

Maintain your shoulders and neck muscles relaxed for the entire exercise.

Raise and lower your leg for ten repetitions before returning to the starting position and repeating to the other side.

3. GLUTES WITH CHAIR

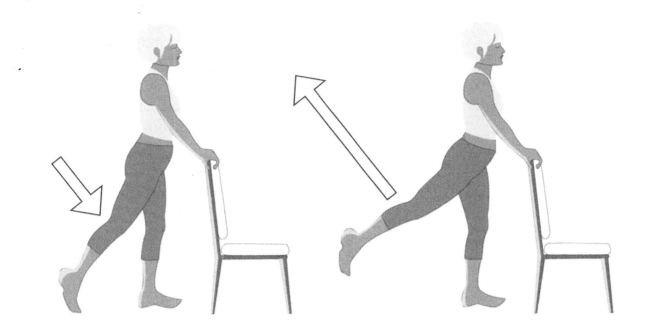

Stand in front of the chair and place both hands on the edge of the chair.

Then, keeping the right leg half bent and the left leg extended, perform backward thrusts with the latter for at least 30 seconds and then proceed with the other.

Repeat the exercise 3 times per each leg.

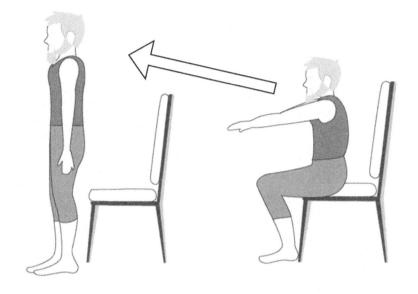

Sit on the edge of the chair.

Put your feet on the ground, hip-width apart, and slightly behind your knees.

Lean forward over your knees and stand up completely without leaning with your hands. Then sit down again. A repetition is done.

Time the time with your watch or mobile phone and repeat this sequence for 1 minute.

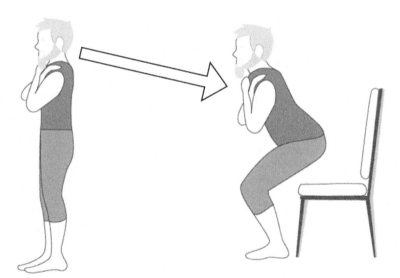

If you don't feel confident enough, use a chair with armrests as a support to get up and sit down.

If a minute is too long, simply write down the number of repetitions of the exercise you were able to do and continue!

If the exercise feels tough ... you can help yourself by crossing your arms in front of your torso, allowing you to lift up.

5. STEP UP

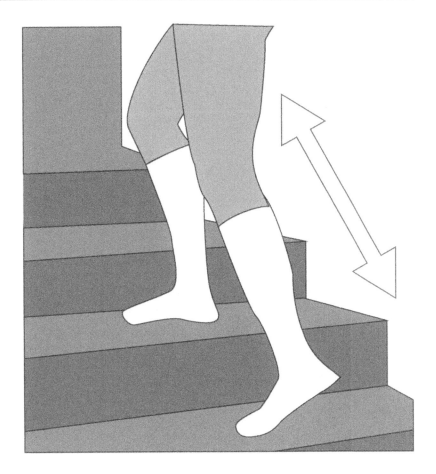

Stand in front of the stairs or a step.

Put your right foot on a step first, and then your left.

Get off doing the same movement but in reverse.

Repeat the exercise 20 times.

If you don't feel confident with your balance, instead of stepping up with both feet one at a time, you can try placing one foot on the step and then returning to the starting position, repeating the movement with the other leg.

This, the most classic of the exercises with the stairs, is ideal for toning the legs and buttocks and can be done with different variations.

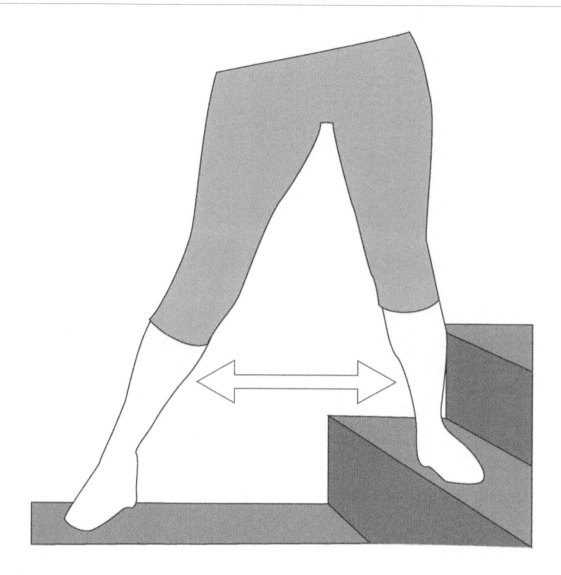

As in the previous exercise, what you want to do now is to position yourself not in front of the stairs but on the side, in parallel.

Then keep your back straight and bring one foot sideways over the step. Return to your normal position, repeating this movement ten times.

When you are done, repeat with the other leg.

POST-ACTIVITY COOLDOWNS

These exercises are great to make your limbs more supple and flexible, and to cool down your body and heartbeat after the exercise.

1. WALL STRETCHING

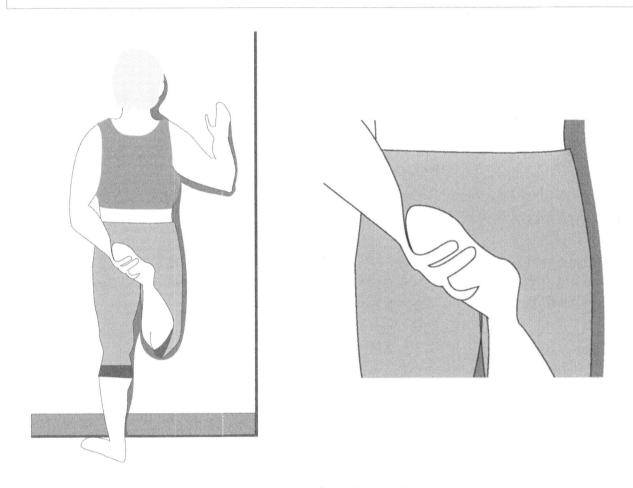

Extensions are very useful for taking care of tired muscles.

In a standing position, simply bring the heel of one leg to the buttock and then, with the hand of the opposite arm, grasp the foot or ankle. It is good to gently pull back and legs so as to work without too much load on the quadriceps.

2. CHAIR STRETCHING

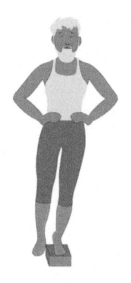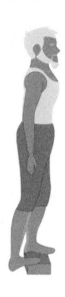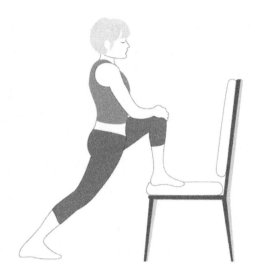

It is useful to identify a support point, such as a wall, a block or a chair, and use them as a support for the cool-down.

For example, you can place one foot so as to lift the leg and bend the knee slightly.
At this point, the pelvis is pushed slightly forward until the inner thigh and groin are slightly tensed. Perfect for preventing tears and pain with ease.

3. HIP AND PELVIS

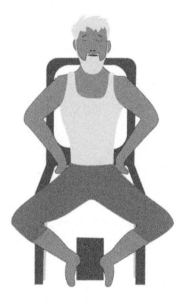

This exercise is very similar to the lotus position in yoga: just position yourself sitting on the chair with your back straight.

Join the soles of your feet together by bending your knees.

Also, with the help of your hands, bring the heels closer and rest them on a support.

4. LIKE A CHILD

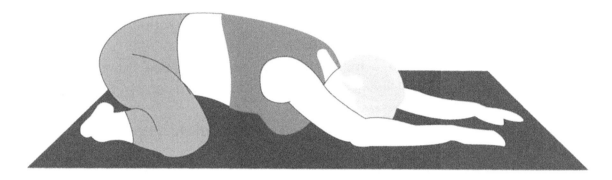

Kneel, bring your big toes against each other, and spread your knees.

Bring the torso towards the ground between the thighs, extend the arms in front of you, but relax the neck and shoulders. Bring your forehead to the ground and leave your elbows bent.

With each exhalation, feel how the pelvis relaxes in the direction of the heels. Observe breathing in your back; imagine a balloon inflating and deflating.

Maintain for at least one and a half minutes.

MAT BEFORE BED (8 MIN)

One of the best stretches that combine flexibility with relaxation are the evening stretching routines to wind down and decompress before bedtime.

In this section, we will use the Yoga mat (you know you will need it sooner or later!). Notwithstanding that, as you will see in the next paragraph, you can stretch before going to sleep directly from the bed!

It's up to you; the result does not change, nor does your restful sleep!

1. PELVIC TILT

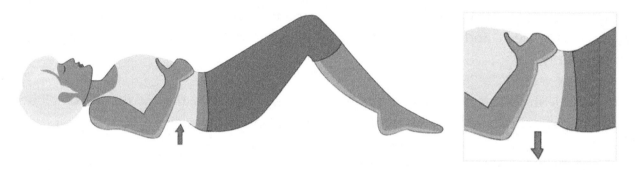

Remain to lie on the mat with the soles of your feet on the mat and slightly apart, your arms at your sides.

Inhale, inflate the abdomen and prepare for movement; exhale, contract the pelvic floor and rise with the pelvis. Inhale and descend; exhale, contract, and lift with the pelvis; inhale and descend, take in good air; exhale, contract, and rise, slightly rotating the coccyx upwards towards the head; inhale and descend.

Do this exercise for about ten repetitions.

2. BRIDGE POSE

Remain to lie on the mat with the soles of your feet on the ground and slightly apart, your arms at your sides.

Inhale, inflate the abdomen and prepare for movement; exhale, contract the pelvic floor and rise with the pelvis.

Instead of going up and down as in the previous exercise, stay up for 20 seconds.

If the exercise feels tough ... you can use a block to be placed in the lumbar area so as not to feel pain.

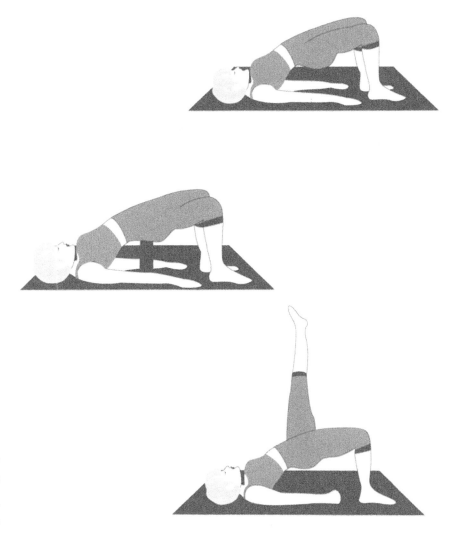

If you feel particularly inspired and can safely perform this movement, finally, you can intensify the position by lifting first one leg and then the other.

Remember not to hold your breath and always keep your stomach in.

Then, vertebra by vertebra, slowly descend onto the mat.

3. ROTATION OF THE HIPS

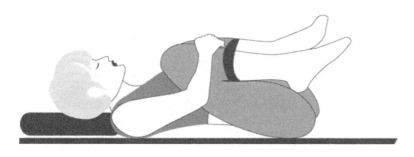

With your hips on the ground, grab your knees and bring your legs to your chest.

Place your hands on your knees and perform clockwise and counterclockwise hip rotations.

This will help you relax and loosen up, but above all, make the pelvic floor elastic and improve the drainage of the lower limbs.

4. GLUTES

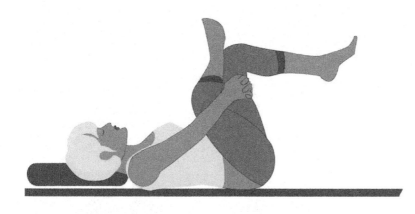

Start by laying on your back. Extend your legs out and put your arms alongside the body.

Now bend the knees, placing the soles of the feet on the mat.

Then cross the right ankle over the top of the right knee as a figure four. Flex the right toes while lifting the left foot off the floor.

Put the right arm through the opening of the legs and clasp the hamstring with both hands.

Make sure the back and head remain flat on the mat. Finally, draw the left shin in towards the body as you press the right knee away from you.

Stay for 20-30 seconds. Repeat to the other side.

5. LEG ON THE SIDE

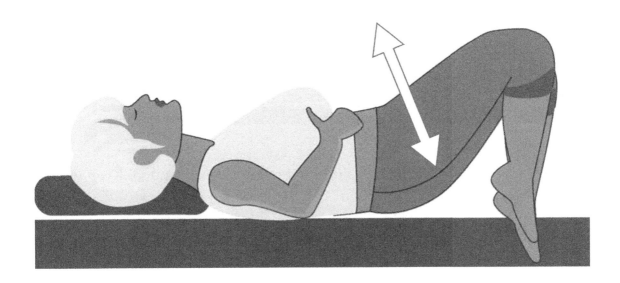

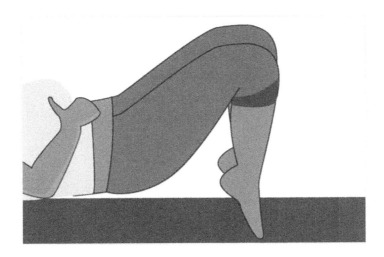

Now bend one knee and touch it with the opposite hand, activating light pressure to bring the knee to the opposite side of the body.

Slowly, lower your hand and legs again and perform on the other side.

Repeat 5-10 times alternately.

6. ADDUCTOR MUSCLES

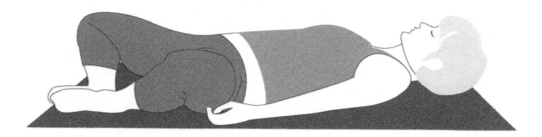

Position yourself on the floor on the mat, sitting with your legs extended. Keep your back straight.

Bring the soles of your feet together, wrapping them with your hands and slowly bringing your knees down. Perform gentle leg swings to encourage a gradual descent by simulating the flapping of butterflies wings.

Open your legs as far as possible, never putting too much strain on the muscles. The goal is to reach the floor with the knees, open the hips fully, and bring the heels as close as possible to the groin area.

Hold the position for 1 to 2 minutes, then inhale and slowly return to the starting position.

7. SAVASANA

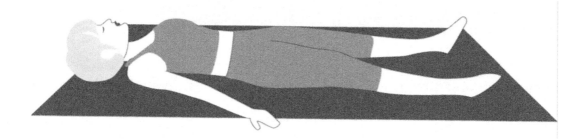

As the name suggests, the Savasana remains perfectly still, in a prone position, with the arms extended along the body and the eyes closed for a sufficient period, not less than 5 minutes, to reach rest, calm and inner peace.

Make sure you don't fall asleep.

At Bed at Night (10 minutes)

1. Breathing

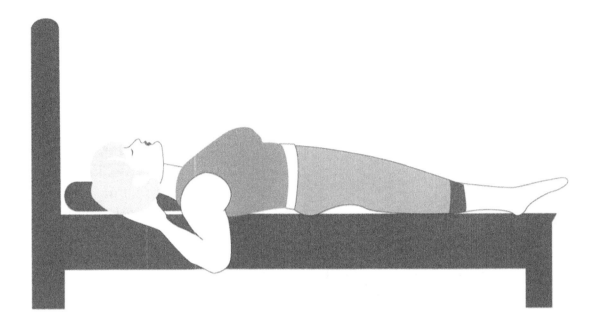

Lie on your stomach with your knees bent and the soles of your feet flat on the bed.

Place one hand on the chest and one on the abdomen. Focus on your breathing. Inhale through the nose, inflating the belly (check with your hands that the abdomen swells while the chest remains stationary). Slowly exhale from your mouth.

Repeat 5-10 times.

From the same position, after inhaling through the nose, perform the same exercise but this time take a short pause holding the air in the lungs and then slowly exhale through the mouth. Repeat five times.

2. GLUTES ON THE WALL

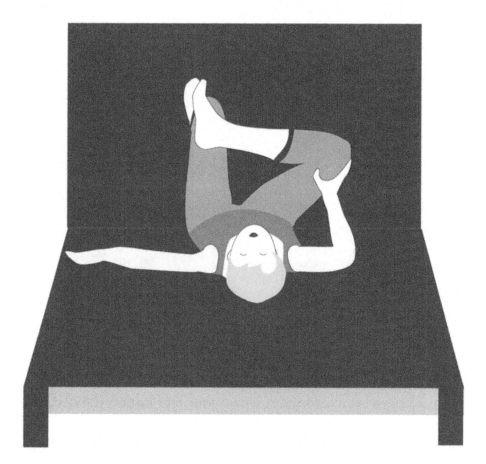

Start by laying on your back, in front of the headboard: your feet will touch the headboard. Then, gently bring your butt close to the wall and lift your legs so that they point high against the wall. Put your arms alongside the body.

Now bend one knees, then cross the right ankle over the top of the right knee as a figure four. Flex the right toes while lifting the left foot off the wall.

Put the right arm through the opening of the legs and clasp the hamstring with both hands.

Make sure the back and head remain flat on the bed. Finally, draw the left shin in towards the body as you press the right knee away from you.

Stay for 20-30 seconds. Repeat to the other side.

3. LEGS UP

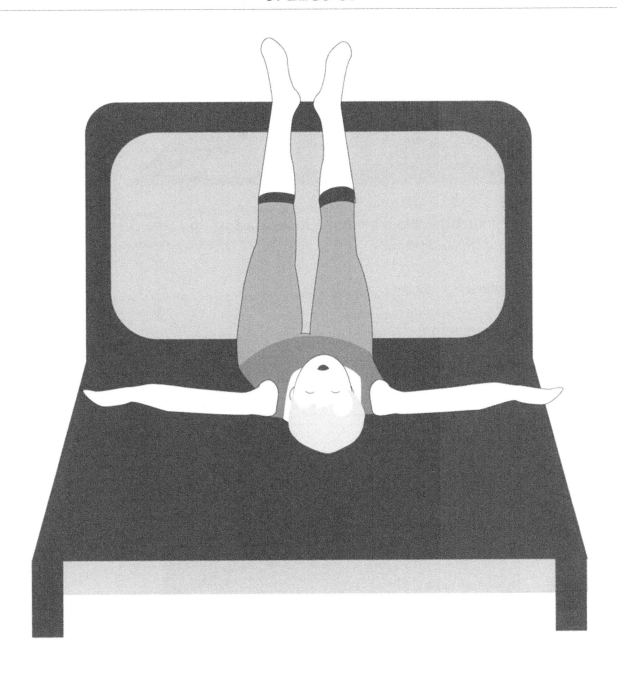

When you have repeated the previous exercise on both the right and left, maintain the position with your feet up on the wall and your back on the bed for at least 1 minute.

4. CRAWLING

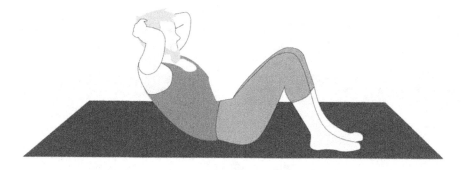

Start by laying on your back. Now bend the knees and try to come closer to them with your torso, activating the abdominals.

Slowly, lower your back.

Repeat 5-10 times alternately.

5. KNEES TO THE CHEST

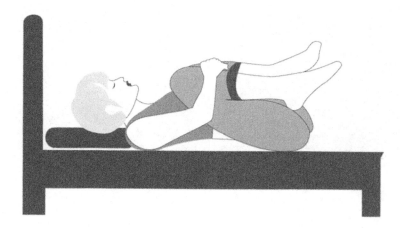

With your hips on the ground, grab your knees and bring your legs to your chest.

Place your hands on your knees and rest for 1 minute.

If you are feeling to, you can perform clockwise and counterclockwise hip rotations.

They will help you relax and loosen up before going to sleep.

Chapter 6
Safe Stretching Routines for Seniors

CLUB N.9 (WITH DUMBBELLS)

Confined at home and without the aid of complicated machinery that in some cases can even be dangerous, you can conduct a series of fairly simple exercises with the help of a chair and small tools (depending on your possibility).

1. BICEPS

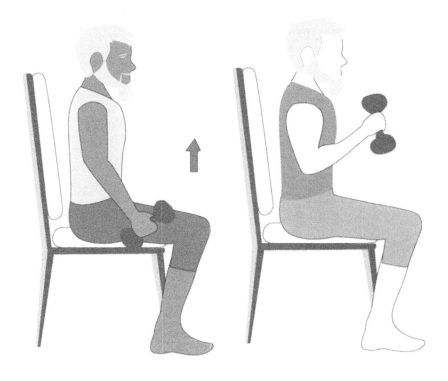

On a chair, sit with your hips back, and you're back firmly against the backrest.

Use a set of dumbbells (we recommend 2-3 kilo weights for beginners).

Begin lifting with your elbows tucked towards your body, lifting towards your chest, until you complete the movement back to the original position.

2. TRICEPS

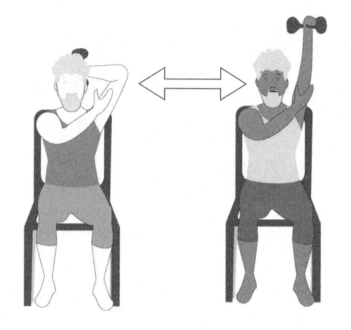

Still sitting on your seat, rest your back against the backrest.

Lift one elbow in the air with a dumbbell and let it fall backward before slowly lifting it above your head, supporting your elbow with the other hand.

Repeat when you have reached the starting position.

3. SHOULDERS

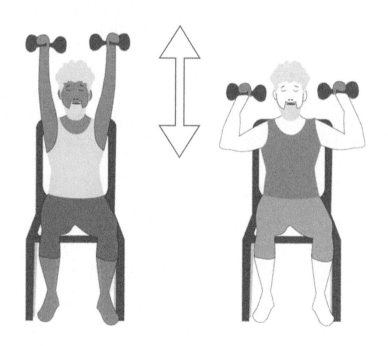

Place your body against the back of the chair, and with a dumbbell in both hands, lift the weights from a 90-degree angle.

As soon as you reach full extension, slowly descend, paying attention.

4. LEGS

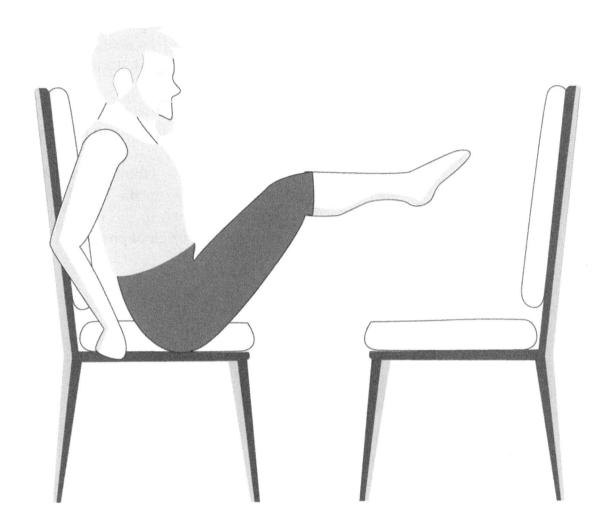

Sitting on the edge of the chair, firmly grasp the sides of the chair with both hands.

Then proceed by extending your legs with the toes pointing upwards.

With the back straight, begin to slowly lift your legs, alternating them as high as possible, before slowly returning to the starting position.

5. TWISTS

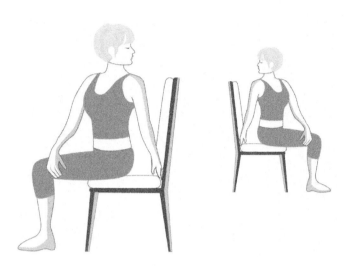

It is great if you practice this exercise with a soft ball (a meditation ball) or other similarly sized object.

While seated, lift your torso's height, keeping it detached from your body.

Then bend the elbows and begin to rotate the torso to the left, then to the center, and then to the right, and then return to the original position.

6. FLEXION OF THE BENT KNEES

While seated, grab the seat of the chair with both hands, move your body forward, making sure that your back is straight, and straighten your legs, making a move until you touch the backrest with your back.

Then slowly raise your legs and pull them towards your body, bending the knees. Slowly lower and return to the starting point.

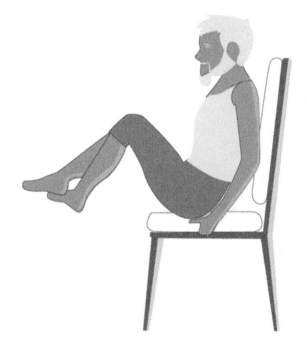

7. KNEES REPS

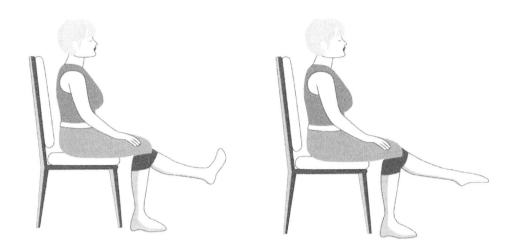

On your chair, lean your back against the backrest, then grasp the sides of the chair with both hands.

Lift one leg in front of you until it is fully extended, then slowly return to the starting position.

Alternate your legs during the exercise.

8. LATERAL STRETCH

Sitting towards the edge of the chair, keep your back straight and feet on the floor.

With the right hand, grab the seat for stability, then raise the left hand towards the ceiling in a curved position.

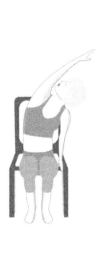
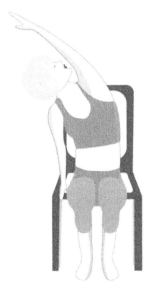

Slowly bend in the direction of the extended arm, and hold for 10-20 seconds.

Return to a straight position and repeat to the other side.

9. HIPS

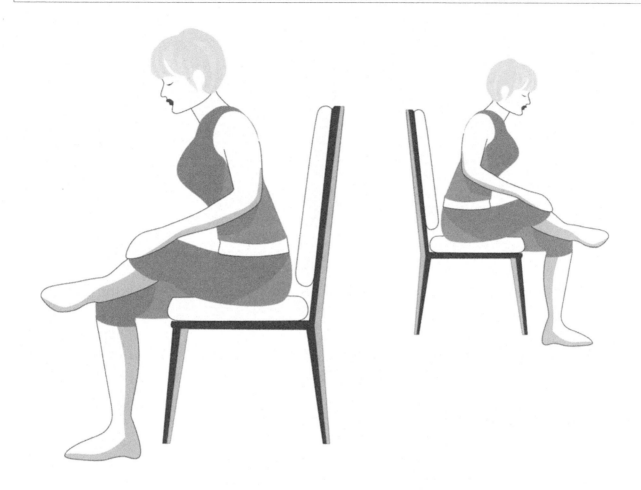

Sit in your chair: your feet flat on the floor.

Maintain your core tight, then cross one leg over the other.

The ankle of the crossed leg has to be extended beyond the leg below.

With your back straight, slowly lean forward as much as possible.

Hold for 10-20 seconds and repeat the operation before alternating with the opposite leg.

THE COMPLETE CYCLE

Doing a full stretch as soon as you get up can provide a lot of energy to the body and release muscle tension for the rest of the day.

You can do it at the beginning, end, or even in the middle of your day. You are free to decide the right time for you. Done before bedtime, however, can help relieve stress and get better sleep (as we previously saw for the other flows).

The crucial thing is to take care of your body through this type of exercise.

1. NECK

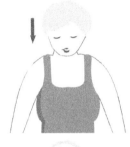
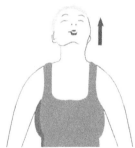

Stand with your arms to the sides of your body. Keep your shoulders relaxed and aligned. Turn your head to the right; hold the position for fifteen seconds.

Look forward again and repeat the movement to the left side.

After this exercise, rest for five seconds and bring your head back without applying force. Hold this position for fifteen seconds, look forward and repeat the movement by tilting your head down for another fifteen seconds.

You can perform the same exercise also while sitting on a chair.

2. SHOULDERS

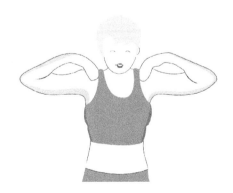

Stand up and, in a slow, careful movement, rotate your right shoulder back.

Repeat the operation ten times.

Now, with the same care, perform the forward rotation motion ten more times.

Repeat the entire procedure with the other shoulder and then with both simultaneously.

3. HIPS AND PELVIS

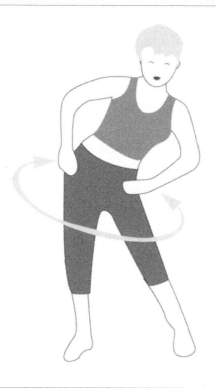

Stand with your legs slightly apart; put your hands on your hips.

Make circular movements clockwise for thirty seconds.

Now, for another thirty seconds, perform the same movements counterclockwise.

4. BACK TWISTS

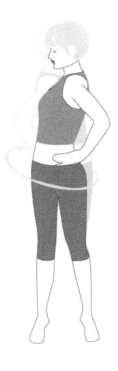

Stand with your legs slightly apart and put your hands on your hips.

Now rotate your torso to the right while keeping your gaze in the direction you are turning.

Return to the starting position; they perform the same movement on the other side.

Do twenty repetitions.

5. LEGS

Start in your standing pose, with your back straight and looking forward.

Gently bring one knee to your chest, supporting it with both hands.

Apply light pressure for fifteen seconds, lower the leg and do the same exercise with the other.

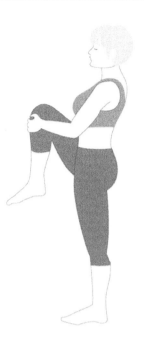

6. FEET

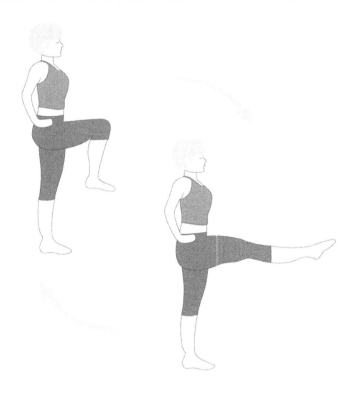

Start in your standing pose with your hands on your hips and your eyes facing forward.

Extend the right leg forward and make circular movements with the foot for ten seconds.

Once this is done, pretend to draw the number '6' in the air with your foot for another ten seconds.

Repeat the exercise with the other leg.

4 DAILY STRETCHES YOU NEED TO DO THEM EVERY SINGLE DAY

1. TORSO STRETCH

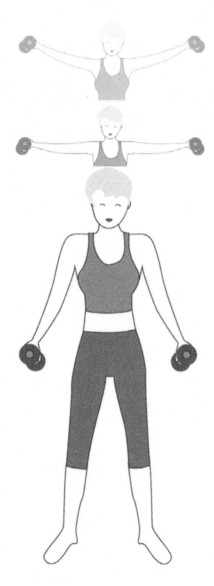

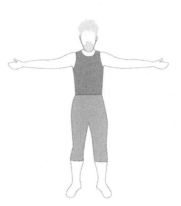

Stand nice and tall. Open up your chest. Shoulders are going back and down at the same time.

Bring your arms open at 45 degrees at the side of the body.

Then, at this very same position, bring them back and open up the chest as much as you can. Squeeze the shoulder blades together and hold here for 20 to 30 seconds. Then shake out your arms to rest.

Then do the exact same exercise, but with your hands open at 90 degrees with the floor. Then shake out your arms to rest.

Following, do the same thing, but with your hands open at 135 degrees with the floor. Then shake out your arms to rest.

Lastly, put your arms up and maintain the stretch for another 30 seconds.
In the end, shake out your arms.

If you feel to, you can also use some light dumbbells.

2. NECK AD CERVICAL

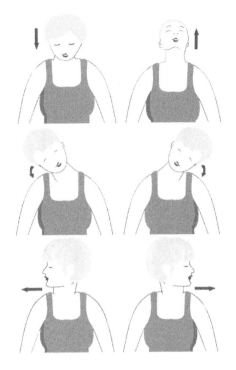

Starting from a sitting position with legs and trunk respectively at 90 ° relative to each other, you can:

•Push the chin inwards for at least 15 seconds and then outwards for 15 seconds. Repeat the movements every three times.

•Make half circles with the head, bringing it to the right towards the shoulder, then towards the chest, and completing towards the left shoulder. Perform the same movement but in reverse. This movement must be repeated ten times in all.

•Make half circles with the head, bringing it to the right towards the shoulder, then looking at the ceiling, and finally towards the opposite shoulder. Perform the same movement but in reverse. This movement must be repeated ten times in all.

•Make complete circles combining the previous exercises, numbers 2 and 3. Perform the total sequence ten times, five clockwise and five counterclockwise.

• Apply light pressure on your head with your left hand, trying to resist with your neck (15 seconds in total). Repeat with the right hand.

3. INNER THIGH STRETCH

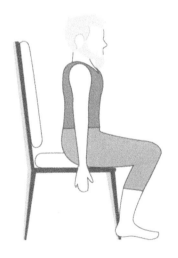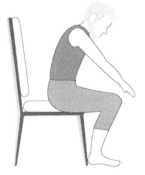

Sit with your legs apart, then tilt your pelvis forward. Keeping your back straight, lean forward as far as you can go.

The knees point upwards; it is possible to activate the feet (hammer-like) or leave them relaxed.

Place your hands on the ground as far forward as possible and support your torso or rest your entire torso on the ground between your legs (advanced level).

Make sure you have warmed up before stretching by doing some light movements.

Hold on to the chair or a wall with your left hand. Bend your right knee.

Grab your leg by the ankle with your right hand and gently pull your foot towards your bottom. Stay in the position for 10 to 20 seconds. Put your leg back down and repeat with your left leg.

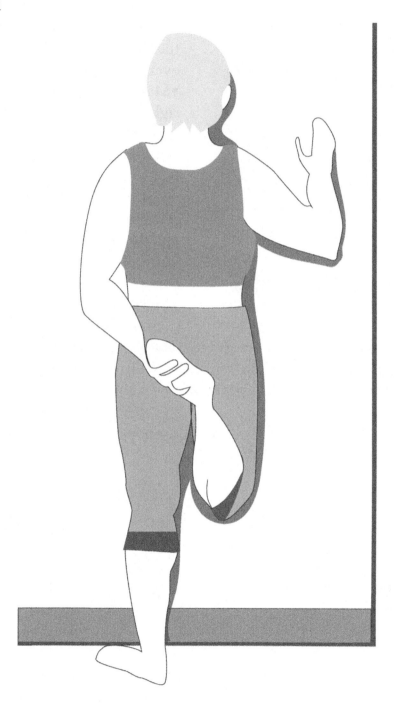

Chapter 7
Get Your Health Back: Muscle Groups and Target Areas

Before proceeding to the exercises for each muscle group, let's talk about how to stay seated correctly in our daily activities.

Daily Posture

Most of us, when sitting, assume a relaxed, slumped position, so the spine resembles a letter C. In other cases, the shape is that of the S when we arch our backs or are tense.

In any case, the 'spoon' position with a curved back and the pelvis detached from the back of the armchair or chair should always be avoided.

It is necessary to position yourself relaxed but with the legs at 90 ° concerning the torso. Slumping on the sofa is another bad habit that compresses the lumbar vertebrae and causes scoliosis and lordosis.

Let's talk about the chair and the table: the chair must be of such a height as not to lean forward to write or work at the desk, and it is good that it is not too far from the work surface.

As we age, it is necessary to purchase, if possible, chairs and armchairs with ergonomic backrests, which allow the body's curves to adapt but maintain the correct posture. And now, let's go straight to the exercises for each targeted area!

EXERCISES FOR THE CERVICAL

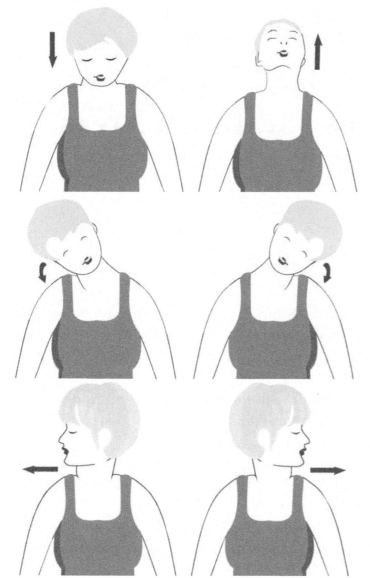

Start from a sitting position with legs and trunk respectively at 90 ° relative to each other.

Push the chin inwards for at least 15 seconds and then outwards for 15 seconds. Repeat the movements every three times.

Make half circles with the head, bringing it to the right towards the shoulder, then towards the chest, and completing towards the left shoulder. Perform the same movement but in reverse. This movement must be repeated ten times in all.

Make half circles with the head, bringing it to the right towards the shoulder, then looking at the ceiling, and finally towards the opposite shoulder. Perform the same movement but in reverse. This movement must be repeated ten times in all.

Make complete circles combining the previous exercises, numbers 2 and 3. Perform the total sequence ten times, five clockwise and five counterclockwise.

Place your left hand on your head, applying light pressure. Try to resist with your neck (15 seconds total). Repeat with the right hand.

HANDS

Start by stretching one arm forward so that it is parallel to the ground, with the palm facing the ceiling. With the other hand, grab the fingers and fold them down.

Hold the position for 15-30 seconds when you feel a pleasant stretch.
Then alternate the arms and do two to four repetitions.

If you can't fully extend your arm, you can do the stretch with your elbow slightly bent.

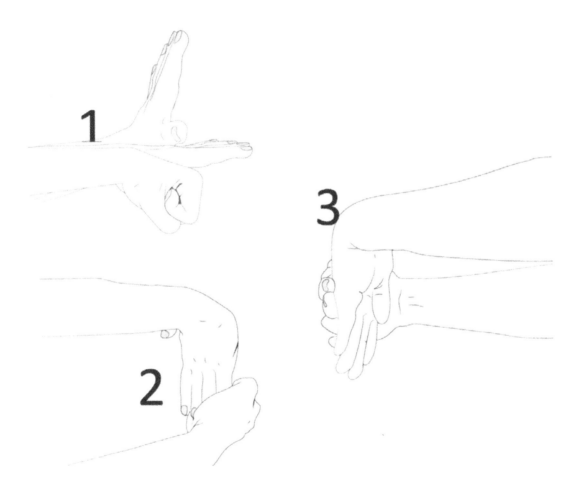

SHOULDERS

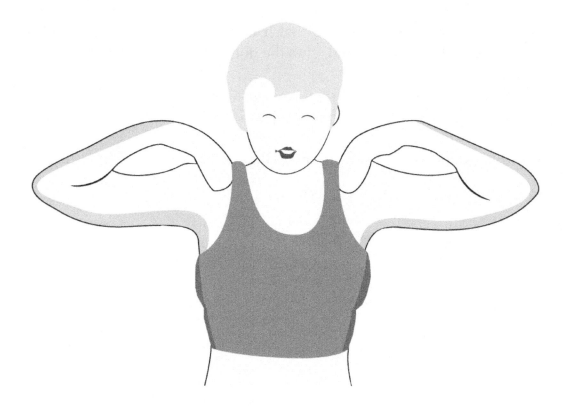

Moving the shoulders is essential to promote mobility and warm the body before the practice.

Sit straight with your chest open and your feet firmly on the floor.

Then slowly, move your shoulders up and down, back and forth, and then proceed with backward rotations.

Breathing from the abdomen with each movement is vital to relax the muscles and prepare us for our practice.

You can use slow exhalations, counting 4 to inhale and 8 to exhale. Gradually increase the number of exhalations to 12 and 16. This system has an immediate calming effect on the nervous system.

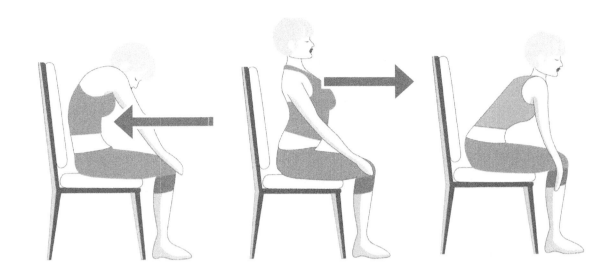

Sit close to the edge of your chair: both feet flat on the floor. Put your hands on your knees or the top of your thighs. Breathe in.

During an inhalation, slowly arch your back, bringing your chest forward and pulling your tailbone and shoulders back.

Then arch the spine by pushing the chest out and as you exhale forcefully, bring the shoulders back to their place and continue like this. Inhale and exhale as you arch your torso downwards.

To exhale, around the back, pull the chest back and the tailbone and shoulders forward. Repeat 3 to 5 times.

LOWER BACK

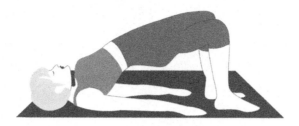

Lie with the soles of your feet on the mat and slightly apart, your arms at your sides.

Inhale, inflate the abdomen and prepare for movement; exhale, contract the pelvic floor and rise with the pelvis. Inhale and descend; exhale, contract, and lift with the pelvis.

Inhale and descend, take in good air; exhale, contract, and rise, slightly rotating the coccyx upwards towards the head; inhale and descend.

Do this exercise for about ten repetitions.

HIP FLEXORS

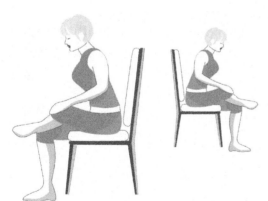

This exercise is amazing for relieving tension in the hips and lower back and irritation of the sciatic nerve.

Start by sitting forward, towards the edge of the chair. Place the right heel on the left knee in a 'four' position. The knee will fall to the right side.

Start gently bending forward until you feel a stretch in your right hip joint. To deepen, gently press the knee down with the elbows. If there is tension or pressure in the knee, back off a little.

For maximum benefit, repeat the pose a second time before continuing.

Make sure to repeat the same sequence on the other side

KNEE

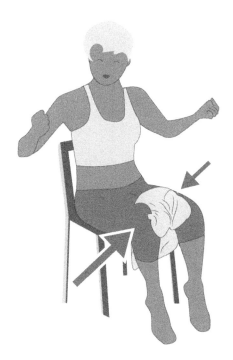

Start by placing a thin but firm pillow between your knees and bring your feet together. Sit straight and keep your legs at a 90-degree angle.

Press your knees strongly together, squeezing the pillow while breathing. Hold for 15 to 20 seconds. Then repeat 3 to 5 times.

Repeat on the second side.

HAMSTRINGS

Stand with one leg extended and your back straight. Put your leg on the chair.

Reach toward your ankle. Keep your knee, neck, and back straight.

The back of your thigh is stretching. Hold for 30 to 60 seconds.

Repeat 2 to 3 times per day.

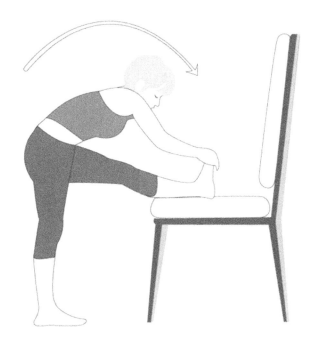

QUADRICEPS

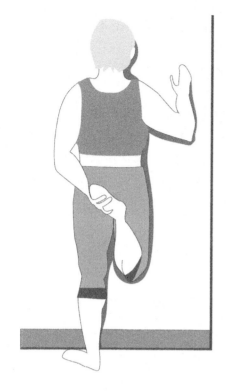

Make sure you have warmed up before stretching by doing some light movements.

Hold on to the chair or the wall with your left hand. Bend your right knee.

Grab your leg by the ankle with your right hand and gently pull your foot towards your bottom. Stay in the position for 10 to 20 seconds.

Put your leg back down and repeat with your left leg.

CALVES

Hold on to a chair, then keep one leg back with your knee straight and your heel flat on the floor.

Bend your elbows and front knee slowly and move your hips forward.

Feel a stretch in the calf.

Stay in the position for 30 to 45 seconds. Then repeat with your other leg.

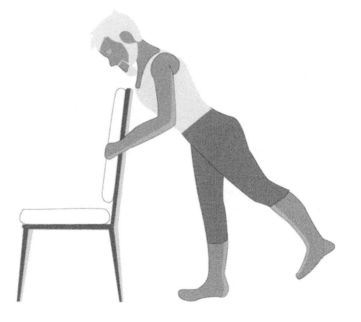

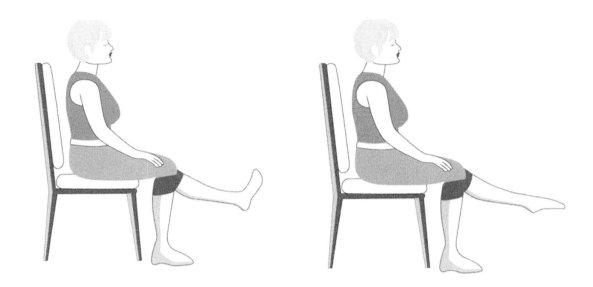

We often underestimate the mobility and strength of our feet, but this is a key factor in maintaining independence and mobility as we age. These exercises can help.

Sit on the chair, your back straight and resting on the backrest and your feet firmly on the ground.

Raise your right leg without exaggerating and start to rotate the ankle clockwise at least five times; stop and make another five rotations counterclockwise.

Now, with your feet back on the ground, lift your left leg, repeating the rotation with the left ankle first in one direction and then in the other.

Return the leg to the starting position and take a few breaths to rest.

When you feel ready, lift your right leg by doing and resume with the ankle rotations, and then switch to the other leg.

Do this at least three/ four times per leg.

Start in your standing pose with your hands on your hips and your eyes facing forward.

Extend the right leg forward and make circular movements with the foot for ten seconds.

Once this is done, pretend to draw the number '6' in the air with your foot for another ten seconds. Repeat the exercise with the other leg.

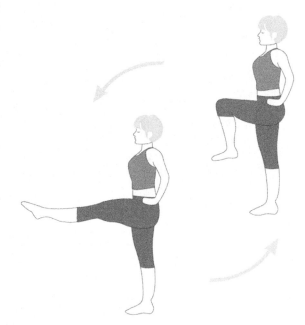

The Bottom Line

Physical activity in the elderly is of fundamental importance, as it develops and improves muscles, bones, and joints. It should never be done by overloading the body but accompanying it in the search for lasting physical well-being over time. The positive effects are also found in mental, as motor activity can be carried out in company, sharing experiences and solutions. Specialists are essential to guide the elderly toward the correct posture and extent of the exercises.

Some gentle gymnastics exercises can sometimes be performed at home, preferably at the beginning, with the supervision of a family member or friend. In any case, consistency is important. Training slows down the physiological decline of the body and is a great way to spend part of the day in good company.

Stretching helps relax the body, lubricate joints, increase range of motion and produce endorphins. Remember to wear comfortable clothes during the exercises and maintain good hydration to avoid injury or muscle cramps. Incorporate stretching into your daily routine, and you will see that the results are guaranteed!

BOOK 3:
CORE AND STRENGTH EXERCISES FOR SENIORS

Chapter 1
Your Inner Power

Physical activity is crucial for living a healthy life both psychologically and muscularly; in recent years, more and more techniques are evolving for movement, introducing training styles that revolutionize the way we see sport and exercise, even for the elderly.

Core stability is among the most exciting techniques which combine breathing and movement. In the following pages, we will examine in more detail what it is and how you can use it to improve your physical and mental condition and prevent aging and injuries due to instability.

It's easy to imagine the types of athletes who focus intensely on core work: boxers, weight throwers, horse riders, skiers... It might surprise you to know that professionals of all kinds find that strengthening the core improves their sports performance. Soccer, softball, and football players need to have a bomb-proof center. And endurance seniors too!

A strong trunk is essential even if you've finished university or worked a long time ago :) because it promotes good posture when you are sitting, walking, or doing strength exercises. It provides the balance to run, jump, dance, or climb stairs to catch the train. If they've ever complimented you on your excellent coordination, you need to thank your core! For people with disabilities, moreover, the trunk sometimes takes responsibility for absorbing imbalances and taking on a more significant part of the force production. Also, the stronger your core, the more immune you become to injury.

As some people say: the Core is You. And I couldn't agree more with them!

As we age, bones weaken, muscle mass and body flexibility decrease, and balance suffers. Combined, these factors can lead to normal daily activities with less agility and, in worst cases, to unexpected and dangerous falls.

To avoid such events as much as possible, it is important to train regularly to keep your physique strong and dynamic.

A decisive role in avoiding falls would be played in particular by the core, the central part of the body between the lower portion of the torso and the lower edge of the pelvis. To keep yourself in shape, there are specific exercises that are easy to do for all ages.

Before investigating further the types of core stability exercises, it is essential to understand what this term means and what it is for.

From a purely scientific point of view, the term core stability identifies the ability of the respiratory diaphragm, abdominal wall, and pelvic floor to stabilize the spine when any movement is made.

This technique is indicated to avoid the potential onset of injuries and pains. Therefore, we can define it as an ideal way of behaving to minimize problems related to sports and physical activity. Incorrect use of core stability leads to various problems in the back, the latter particularly vulnerable and predisposed to degeneration in correspondence with impetuous and wrong movements.

When we approach core stability, we refer to all the muscles of the abdominal-lumbopelvic complex, incorporating a double musculature, the deep one and the external one. In the first case, the muscles have the task of giving stability to the spine and pelvis, while in the second case, the muscle band monitors the movement of the limbs subject to gravity and external loads.

Wanting to give it a simpler purpose to interpret, we can say that the core is responsible for stabilizing the movement of the pelvis and chest, favoring the expulsion of waste in the muscles.

Chapter 2
Core Training: Boost for Your Health

What are the advantages and benefits of having a strong core? Core stability is very important in daily life as it brings various benefits to those who adopt it.

They are the muscles that ensure that our spine can move safely and allow us to maintain correct posture. The action of these muscles enables our body, particularly our spine, to deal with the imbalances generated by the forces that come into play during movement. In particular, the action of the transverse abdominal muscle should be emphasized, a power that creates a band around the waist and that, more than any other, contributes to the spine's stability at the lumbosacral level, especially when there is a poor balance situation of our body.

The main importance, moreover, is alleviating back pain, that is, all those problems related to the back of the body, particularly subject to a load of muscles and bones.

It is essential to analyze the benefits individually to have a clearer examination of the importance of core stability. Specifically, the concrete benefits are verified for posture, lumbar problems, spine, knees, and sports performance.

Improving posture

Incorrect posture significantly impairs the right balance between body and mind. Postural pain and the consequences in the medium to long term can significantly affect people's health. Core stability allows you to fight incorrect posture and have the right postural behavior during the day.

Many underestimate the importance of correct posture, eventually finding themselves with severe back and neck pain. Being able to better manage the posture over the years guarantees a healthier life physically, but above all, that gives well-being to the psychological component. The body will automatically behave in the best way to protect the muscles through proper breathing, movement, and muscle training.

Helping solve lower back problems

Especially in people with a sedentary lifestyle, lower back pain is one of the most common problems. About 90% of people suffer from this pathology at least once, causing inflammation to induce users to intervene with physiotherapy. One of the advantages of core stability is the concrete reduction of pain when suffering from lumbar problems, guaranteeing a feeling of immediate relief with which to continue the working or sports day without any thought.

Vertebral column relief

When you have lower back problems, other areas of the body are most likely affected; one of the most recurrent problems is that inherent to the spine. Taking a wrong position during daily activities or not having an adequate posture can lead to scoliosis or lordosis, which is certainly not pleasant. Core stability takes care to induce users to behave appropriately to minimize problems of this entity, freeing the subject from potential physiotherapy treatments and annoying back pains.

Knees relief

Thanks to the core stability, it is possible to eliminate all those damages related to the knees. Especially at a certain age, many people, after a lifetime of walking the wrong way, run into severe pain in their knees. Although there is a deterioration of the cartilage due to age in many cases, the pain is due to inappropriate posture in many others. Prevention, in this case, is essential to feel good about your body

Chapter 3
Core: Let's Take a Closer Look

In the previous chapters, we have anticipated the areas involved for core stability, but what are the muscles that belong in detail to this process?

Commonly speaking, we mean the 'core of the body', which is an area between the lower portion of the torso and the lower edge of the pelvis.

The core is given considerable importance in the functional expression of movements, as it could be defined as the first ring of any kinetic chain. For this reason, a possible lack of muscular trophism and being responsible for lower athletic performance can imply various muscle-joint imbalances and predispose the onset of injuries.

Many centuries ago, Yoga had already identified the importance of the core and its functioning for health and quality of life. On the other hand, in the West, these concepts were only understood at the turn of the twentieth century, thanks to the Pilates discipline. Today, core development is integral to athletic sports, fitness or wellness, and preventive and rehabilitative physical training.

The main muscles of the core reside in the abdomen, waist, middle and lower back, and hips. Let's go into more detail.

It is necessary to divide two types of muscles, internal and external, that have different functions:
- as for the internal muscles, those that belong to the core are the diaphragm, pelvic muscles, multifidus muscles, internal obliques, and transverse abdominal muscles;
- the external muscles involved are the quadrate loin, erector spine, external oblique, and straight abdominal muscles.

The muscles, in this case, are essential to moving safely and always having a correct posture. When imbalances arise, it would be essential to have muscles ready to rebalance internal and external forces so as not to create friction or injury to the most important parts of the body.

So, the main muscles of the core are:

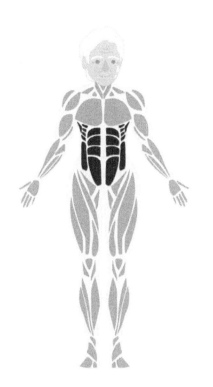 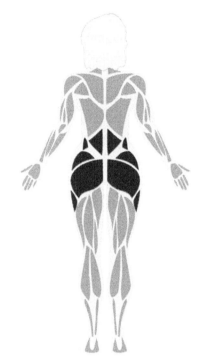

- all of the pelvic floor;
- transverse abdomen;
- multifidus;
- internal and external obliques
- rectus abdominis;
- spinal erectors (sacrospinal);
- diaphragm.

Although they play a less central role, they can also be considered core:
- the lumbar - deep portion of the square of the loins;
- deep rotators;
- cervical muscles;
- rectus anterior and lateral of the head;
- long neck;
- great dorsal;
- gluteus maximus;
- trapezoid.

Note: Not everyone agrees on the relevance of many of the muscles mentioned. It should be specified that those most involved reside, as anticipated in the introduction, between the abdomen and the pelvis.

Chapter 4
Core Training: Essential for Seniors

Continuing to have a strong core even when you are living your senior years is important because this muscle group, representing the connection point between the upper and lower body, is responsible for most of the movements necessary to lead a satisfying life.

Training the core, therefore, is a priority, which amplifies even more after the age of 50: it is at that age that the body begins to weaken, making a more intelligent contrasting action necessary.

In addition to preventing injuries, a more robust midsection helps improve body stability and coordination, counteract back pain, and improve posture and daily movements.

Static core function

The core's static function is its core's ability to align and stabilize the skeleton to withstand a specific force.

A case in point of the static core function is 'firing a rifle' from the prone position - lying on the stomach. To maintain maximum accuracy, the shooter must be able to transfer his body weight and rifle to the ground. Any attempt by the shooter to move the line of fire (moving the sight on the target with the arms rather than following the movement with the whole body) would fail. To maintain a maximum level of accuracy, one should not simply exert muscle force on the rifle but focus on the axis of the skeleton for stabilization. The core, resting on the ground and relatively far from the rifle, stabilizes the spine and pelvis, creating an advantage for the shoulder, arms, and neck. For the peripheral elements to remain as still as possible, without moving unnecessarily, the spine, pelvis, and rib cage must be aligned.

Therefore, it is possible to say that the core muscles provide support to the axial portion of the skeleton (skull, spine, and coccyx) by stabilizing the upper part and, thus, the rifle.

Dynamic core function

The nature of the dynamism takes into account both the skeletal structure and the external resistance; consequently, it affects both the muscles and the joints differently than the static position.

For this reason, during dynamic movement, the component of central muscular contraction is higher than that of skeletal 'rigidity,' instead more important in staticity. This is because the purpose of the contraction is not to oppose a static, immutable resistance but to resist a force that changes on the plane of movement. During movement, the body segments must fluidly absorb resistance; therefore, the tendons, ligaments, muscles, and innervations play different and changing roles. These include postural reactions to changes:

• of speed (rapidity of a contraction);
• of movement (reaction time);
• power (amount of stamina won over a while).

A simple example of a dynamic core function is walking on a mountain path. In this case, the body should resist gravity while moving in a specific direction, balancing itself despite the irregularities of the ground. This forces a balanced alignment of the central axis and the extremities and simultaneously supports the momentum by pushing from the ground in the opposite direction. It is generally believed that the lower limbs are primarily responsible for walking and running, but this is not the case. The 'main engine' is the core, on which the thighs and legs can develop propulsion.

All being said, limiting ourselves to this is not enough. To keep fit as the years go by, it's also crucial to add at least a routine of moderate aerobic activity per day (10 minutes are enough, don't worry) to your fitness routine. But I got you covered: that why you are here!

Chapter 5
How Do You Train the Core?

Core training must contain a combination of strength, flexibility, and control. Training must therefore be functional. In essence, the goal is to provoke and test the responsiveness of the 'center' of our body to external stimuli through isometric, static, or moving exercises, and also thanks to the use of tools that stimulate balance and coordination skills.

Following this information, I intend to sensitize you on how useful it is to strengthen and strengthen this area, starting from straightforward and practical exercises.

From here and after that, an infinite world of progressive workouts opens up to challenge and stimulate the core to the maximum, exercises that can only be performed after reaching a remarkable degree of conditioning, perception, and activation.

My advice is always to rely on a professional in the sector, at least in the approach phase, to help you enhance the sensations and benefits.

Get involved, work on the core, strengthen your inner power and live a happier life. It's just as simple!

What NOT to do

Core training has often been reduced to just exercising the abdominal muscles and extending the spine to work the lower back muscles. In these analytical exercises in which the spinal column is kept still, we activate the central area of the body and consequently strengthen them... but at what cost?

Changing the physiological curves of the back with this type of exercise generates unnecessary stress that can cause various spine pathologies. The repeated flexion movement produces tension in the lower part of the fibrous ring. It can consequently cause a herniated disc, and/or the disc is crushed and compresses some nerves in the lumbosacral complex.

On the other hand, the extension movements of the spine can damage the joints, generating lumbar arthritis or osteoarthritis.

So, in an ideal training program, in addition to the exercises to be performed, it is essential to know the mistakes to avoid.

An exercise performed poorly can lead to more problems than an exercise aimed at a muscle band that you do not want to improve. What are the errors to be ruled out during physical activity?

Stretching and warm-up

One of the most common mistakes of those who practice physical activity is to skip stretching completely. As the exercises that will be performed also have the function of awakening the muscles and internal organs, it is advisable to carry out the stretching after the core and strength training, to avoid injuries due to the cold or sudden movements.

Speed of execution

Many people, taken by the desire to reduce back pain, perform the exercises too quickly. The success of an exercise, especially of core stability, passes through the perfect execution of the movements. Slow moving is definitely a better condition for the awakening muscles, which can be speeded up when fully active.

Accessories to use

Some core exercises take advantage of dedicated accessories for better movement execution.

There are many tools on the market to add to your core training; still, it is very important to know how to choose them for their physical activity.

An accessory that is disproportionate in weight and functionality can lead to more problems than solutions, invalidating a job that must be performed correctly to not inflame the muscle groups. Core stability professionals can recommend the accessories suitable for your training program.

In conclusion, core work should be achieved with exercises that involve muscular work to stabilize the spine, causing instability with external loads, and not with activities that involve movement of the spine.

The best options for doing the core work actively, therefore, are functional training and the plank, in which movement is produced in the most distant body segments, in particular in the shoulder-blade joint and the pelvis joint.

With functional exercises, the contraction of the core muscles is sought by generating unilateral instability, both through traditional weights and by exploiting gravity.

Training as a senior

Older people can perform specific exercises to strengthen the abdominals and other stabilizing muscles of the trunk and pelvis to improve their body balance. This translates into a better protective function of the spine, an improved posture, and a greater ability to perform more or less complex movements both during sports and in everyday life.

For this purpose, I have devised a real Core Training, simple and effective exercises to train the core muscles or the main stabilizing muscles of the pelvis and trunk, including the abdominals (straight abdominal, obliques, and transverse).

Good joint stability allows for adequate motor control and optimal force application during daily activities such as climbing or descending stairs, picking up an object from the ground, ironing, etc.

In short, core stability exercises serve to:

• Strengthen the abdomen, buttocks, and back;

• Improve balance (hence the name 'core stability');

• Prevent back pain and injuries even in old age.

However, it is good practice to consult your doctor before performing the exercises listed below. Here are the most suitable exercises to strengthen the core after age 50.

Chapter 6
Warm-Up

Is warm-up really important for training? What effects does it have on our body? Does it always have to be accompanied by stretching in the preparatory phase?

Almost always, those who practice any physical activity neglect or attach little importance to warming up, which is, on the contrary, the crucial phase of every workout, useful for guaranteeing the right approach, physical and mental, to performance, be it amateur or professional. The reason for the lack of interest? It is believed that it is not very useful and boring compared to the sporting activity to which it is connected.

However, 'warm-up' literally serves to raise the heat, the body temperature, by one or two degrees with beneficial purposes for the whole organism, especially before core and strength training. Mainly it improves blood fluidity by promoting oxygenation of the muscles and their elasticity to avoid contractures, strains, or tears.

The 'cold' muscle runs the risk of shortening too suddenly as it is not ready for the gesture to be performed or of stretching excessively when not warmed up. Bringing oxygen to the muscles also means returning energy that can be spent during activity, which translates into an improvement in performance, as the increase in temperature promotes blood circulation and, consequently, the elasticity of the muscles and tendons.

In practice, what does warm-up prevent? It prepares muscles, tendons, and ligaments to approach exercise correctly, improves performance, and prevents injuries when performed with logic.

It is also essential both to safeguard the musculoskeletal system from potential trauma and to activate the cardio-circulatory system and the body's physiological functions.

At the joint level, the increase in temperature results in an increase in the production of synovial fluid, which guarantees the lubrication of the joints, gradually favoring a greater range of motion.

In general, during a good warm-up, there is a metabolic activation and an intensification of the activity of the cardiovascular system, which predisposes the body to better physical performance.

The activity usually practiced to start the warm-up phase is a slow run, even on the spot, because it sets in motion a large part of the muscles without the risk of trauma.

So, it is really useful to perform a targeted warm-up, adding exercises that specifically stress the parts of the body that will be most challenged by the training performance you are about to face.

One last important tip before starting: don't stretch before training.

This activity must only follow the exercise routine because practicing it first causes tension in the muscles, which reduces blood flow and increase oxidation.

Before starting training, therefore, it is important to perform an easy and short warm-up to stimulate the activity of the body. For example:

• walking / running on the spot;
• lifting your knees while walking in place;
• walking through the house.

Valid alternatives can be using an exercise bike or bicycle, swimming performed slowly, or even walking at a fast pace.

Exercises in isometry or repetitions?

Isometry is static muscle contraction training. The term 'isometric,' after all, combines the Greek words 'Isos' (equal) and 'metric' (measure); it means that in these executions (for example, a core training exercise), the length of the muscle and the joint angle do not change, although the force of contraction can vary significantly.

Unlike the exercises with repetitions, therefore, isometry allows you to train the core without movements but only by maintaining the position for a predetermined amount of time.

One of the simplest examples of understanding isometry is the execution of the front plank.

The main advantage of choosing isometric exercises is that you can do them anywhere, only using your body weight in support.

The sitting exercises are even more practical, versatile, and ideal for rehabilitation and for seniors.

In our case, the same advice always applies: choose the method and exercises for which you are ready and for which your body is ready. Don't take the initiative without consulting your doctor and trainer, but don't put limits on what you can learn on the journey of core and strength training!

GETTING READY

For effective core ad strength training, performing various exercises with the circuit training method is advisable. This method consists of fluidly passing from one exercise to another, like a real 'circuit.'

As a beginner, 8-15 repetitions per exercise/pose are sufficient for maintaining a static-isometric position for about 30 seconds or up to 1 minute.

Performing at least 3-6 laps of the circuit is advisable. The fatigue limit can be estimated on the ability to perform each rep 'cleanly.'

Finally, I always recommend wearing comfortable, breathable, and elastic clothing to perform the exercises as smoothly as possible.

And get a towel to use to wipe away sweat or place it on the mat.

These following exercises can address the whole body and can be performed even when there is little space available. Let's find out!

FIRST THING FIRST: BREATH

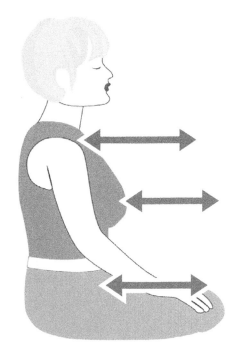

Breathing is a natural physiological function that allows us to obtain the oxygen necessary for our body. When practicing a sport, knowing how to breathe correctly helps to improve performance and allows you to achieve maximum results in terms of physical well-being.

The most suitable breathing is diaphragmatic breathing, which children know well, but which adults sometimes tend to forget. With thoracic breathing, at chest height, shallow breathing is carried out, which brings less oxygen to the body. The consequence is the feeling of needing to breathe sooner than necessary.

Therefore, a correct breathing technique is essential during training, when metabolism increases and, consequently, energy consumption.

Before training, therefore, prepare your breath for the exercise session.

Take five deep breaths, inhale through the nose, swell the belly and diaphragm, and exhale through the mouth slowly. In this way, your body will be prepared to face training, and you will feel more relaxed at the same time.

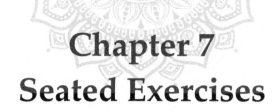

Chapter 7
Seated Exercises

Exercises for Beginners

SEATED TWISTS

Sit firmly on a chair and place your feet on the ground in front of you. Bring your arms to your chest and lean back as comfortably as possible.

As you engage your core muscles, rotate your torso to the left.

From the starting position, repeat the sequence of movements on the right side.

Complete three sets of fifteen repetitions each.
If you can't reach that number, stop before the effort becomes too much.

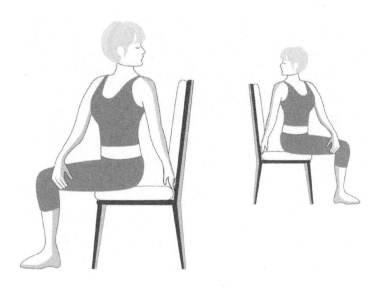

CURL ON A CHAIR

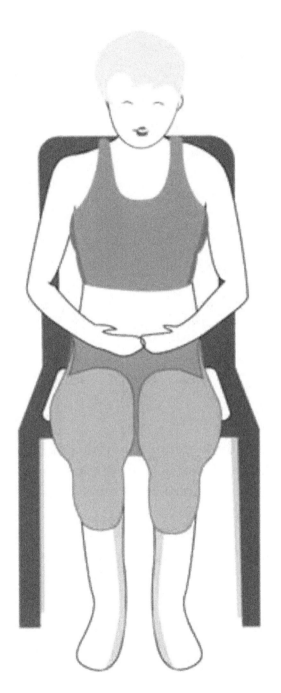

Sit on a chair, placing your feet firmly on the ground and contracting your core muscles and abdominals for at least one minute.

Keep the spine straight while inhaling and bringing the head back.

Stop just before touching the backrest, exhaling as you return to the starting position.

Perform two sets of five repetitions each.

ABDOMINAL VACUUM

The stomach vacuum is a gymnastic exercise to tone the abdominal belt with breathing. It is based on it and does not require any tools. When done regularly, it helps tone deeper abdominals such as the transverse muscle and have a flat stomach within a few weeks.

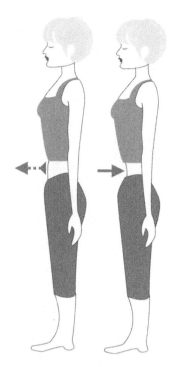

This exercise is inspired by a yoga technique called Uddiyana Bandha, becoming famous thanks to bodybuilders like Arnold Schwarzenegger, Frank Zane, and Ronnie Coleman. They have introduced this core activation into their routine for reaching the abdominal tortoise. The transverse muscle brings the viscera in and is essential for having core stability and a correct posture.

It is, therefore, an exercise within everyone's reach: those with back or neck problems, men and women, elderly, sports and sedentary people! Coordinate breathing and contraction of the abdominals, and that's it!
Moreover, performing the abdominal vacuum daily helps you dispose of stress and oxygenate the body and brain.

Also called 'ventral breathing,' this technique calms the vegetative nervous system (i.e., the body's automatic functions: digestion, respiration, arterial and venous circulation, etc.). The more you train it, the more you increase the intra-abdominal pressure and protect your spine from damage.

The transverse is easily trained by the voluntary movement of pushing the belly in and, forcing exhalation, throwing the air out.

Contrary to classic abdominal exercises that strain the spine and neck and can cause muscle problems, abdominal breathing has no impact on the back.

To perform this type of exercise, you want to inhale and contract your abdomen, sending your belly as deep as you can. Hold for a few breaths and then release through exhalation.
Repeat 3 times.

EXERCISES FOR ADVANCED

SCISSORS

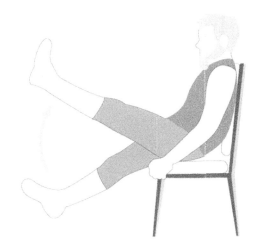

Sitting on the edge of the chair, firmly grasp the sides of the chair with both legs.

Then proceed by extending your legs with the toes pointing upwards, trying to keep your back straight.

Inhale and pull your belly in, then begin to slowly lift your legs, alternating them as high as possible, before slowly returning to the starting position.

BOAT POSE

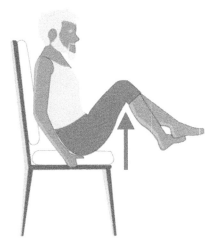

Start by sitting in the mat or chair with your knees facing forward and your feet flat on the floor.

Move to the edge of the chair; lean back slightly, and place your hands behind you on the chair.

As you exhale, lift your feet off the floor and bring your knees towards your chest. During the entire process, keep your back straight and engage your abdominal muscles

If you find this posture simple, you can also add balance to the pose by lifting your arms close to your legs.

Continue to breathe deeply while holding this position for 30 seconds to one minute. To release, slowly lower your feet to the floor and sit straight.
Repeat two or three times, never forgetting to breathe deeply!

Chapter 8
Standing Exercises

EXERCISES FOR BEGINNERS

SQUATS

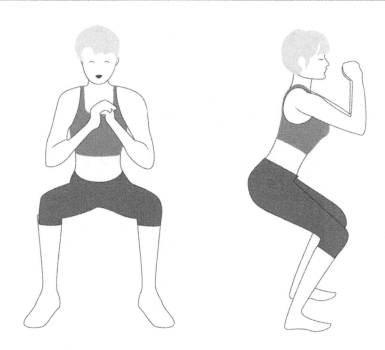

Stand upright, with legs apart, feet turned slightly outward, and hands resting on thighs. You can use a wall behind you if it's more comfortable.

Then bend the knees while keeping your back straight. Stop before the buttocks reach the level of the knees.

Exhale and return to the starting position.
Perform three sets of ten repetitions each.

LATERAL LEG RAISES

Standing erect with feet together and hands on hips.
As you lift your left leg to the side, exhale and return to the starting position.

Keep the trunk and shoulders aligned throughout the movement by contracting the abdomen.

Maintain unaltered curves of the spine. Stabilize the supporting leg by contracting the buttocks and abdomen.

Perform all repetitions, then repeat with the right leg.

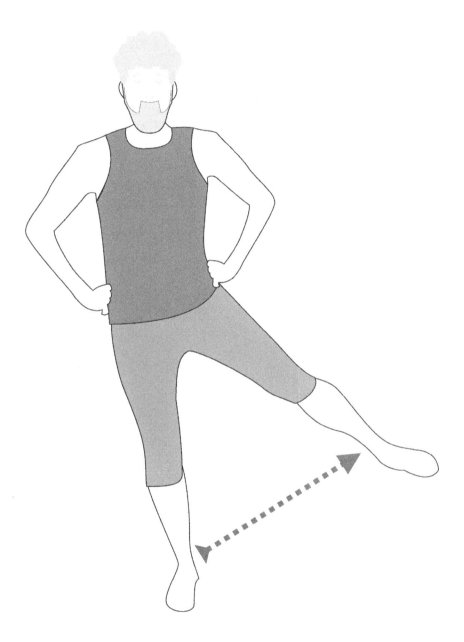

FRONT LEGS RAISE

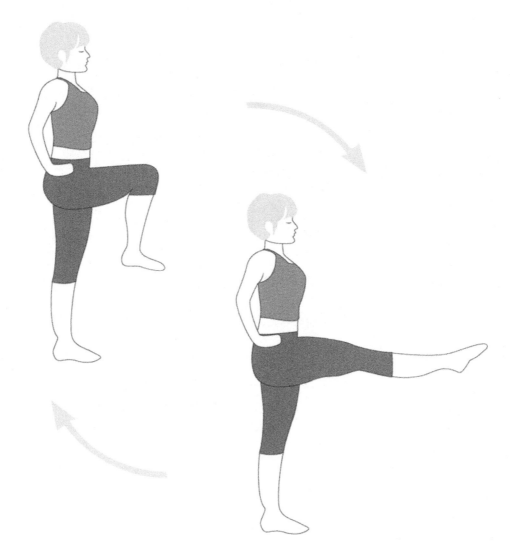

Start from a standing position. Keep both feet on the ground and arms at your hips for balance.

Lift the right knee upwards as far as possible, then lower the foot to the ground.

Maintain unaltered curves of the spine.

Stabilize the supporting leg by contracting the buttocks and abdomen.

Perform all repetitions, then repeat with the left leg.

EXERCISES FOR ADVANCED

HALF LUNGES

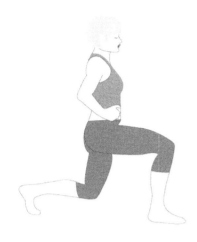

Stand upright, keeping your feet together and your arms at your sides.

Step forward and bend your left leg to form a right angle.

From the starting position, repeat the same movement on the other side.

Distribute your body weight evenly between the right and left foot. The back, shoulder, hip, and knee should be aligned in the lunge position.

Do three sets of ten repetitions each.

STANDING CROSSBODY KNEE DRIVE

Pull your belly back towards your spine from a standing position, with your feet shoulder-width apart and your hands behind your ears.

Use the core to lift the left knee and rotate the body until it meets the right elbow. Lower the leg.

Return to the starting position. Alternate sides with each repetition.

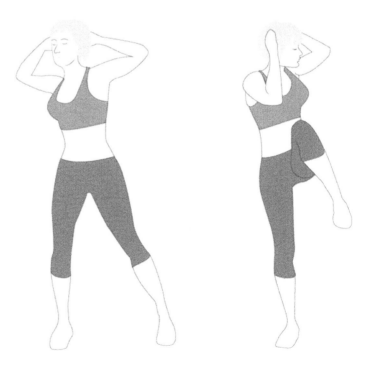

TOY SOLDIERS

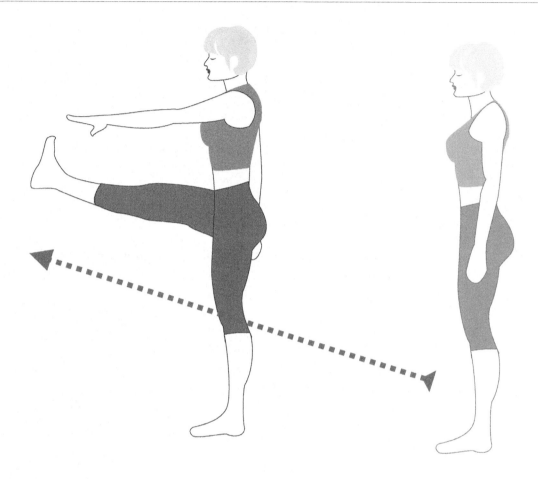

Start with a standing position: cross your arms in front of you.
Bring the rib cage in and strengthen the core by pulling the navel towards the spine and keeping the pelvis relaxed.

To maintain balance, lift your left leg to keep it as straight in front of you as possible, using your core to keep from losing your position.

Lower the leg slowly, keeping the middle part of the body in traction.

Alternate legs with each repetition.

This exercise is excellent for improving the hamstrings' flexibility and mobility and working on the core muscles.

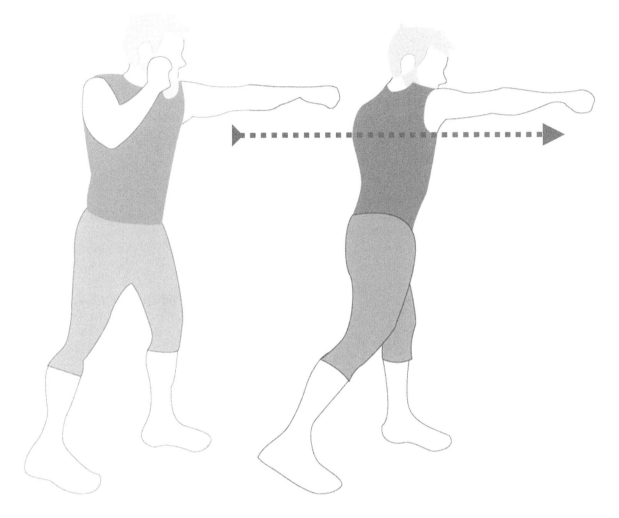

From a standing position, keep your feet shoulder-width apart.

Bring the rib cage in and strengthen the core by pulling the navel towards the spine and keeping the pelvis in traction.

Extend your arms alternately, punching the air imaginary, alternating sides, and gradually increasing the pace.

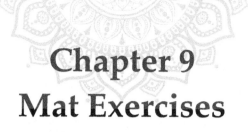

Chapter 9
Mat Exercises

EXERCISES FOR BEGINNERS

BIRD DOG OR QUADRAPLEX

It stimulates the core, balance, and coordination, and it is performed 'face down'.

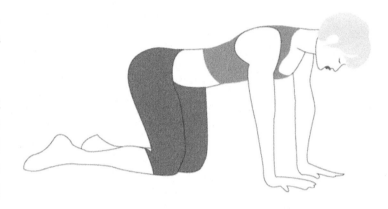

In the quadrupedal position, on the hands and mat, with the back parallel to the floor, extend one arm forward and the contralateral leg back, pointing outward.

It is an exercise that can be done in isometry or alternating repetitions on both sides.

Make sure not to lower your hips and shoulders and arch your back.

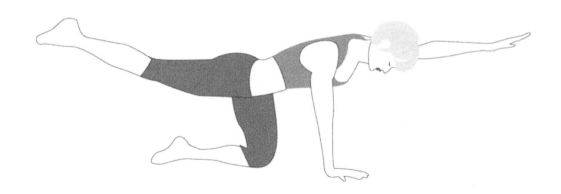

PRONE FLUTTERS

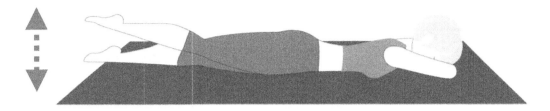

This pose mainly recruits the multifidus muscles in the lower back that play a vital role in stabilizing the spine.

From the prone position, with your arms stretched above your head, or crossed under your forehead, raise your right arm and left leg at the same time, then slowly lower them. You can also keep your hands under your forehead and lift one foot at a time.

Repeat with the opposite arm and leg and continue alternating.

It is an exercise that can be done in isometry or alternating repetitions on both sides.

KNEELING REAR LEG RAISE

On the mat, get in the 4-legged position and make sure your weight is evenly distributed on each point.

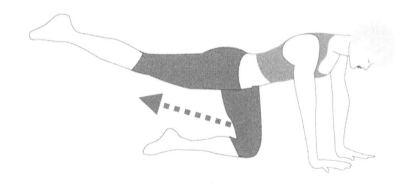

While engaging your core, extend your right leg back so that it hovers slightly above the ground.

Keeping your leg straight, lift it as high as possible without arching your back or feeling pain. Lower and return to the starting position.

Repeat the sequence of movements on the other side.

Perform three sets of ten repetitions each.

GLUTE BRIDGE

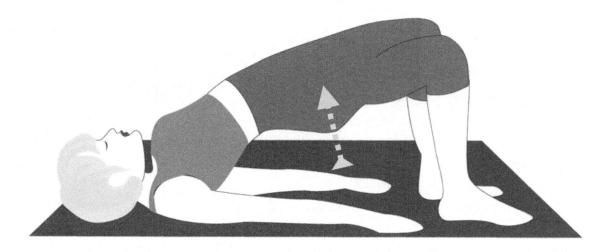

Lie on the mat on your back and bend your knees; feet flat on the floor, positioned hip-width apart.

Push your lower back to the ground and contract your abdominal muscles.

As you exhale, lift your hips off the floor until you form a diagonal line from the knees to the rib cage.

Do not over-stretch your hips to avoid damaging your lower back. Press your heels to the floor to keep yourself stable.

Inhale and return to the starting position.
Perform ten repetitions.

CRUNCH

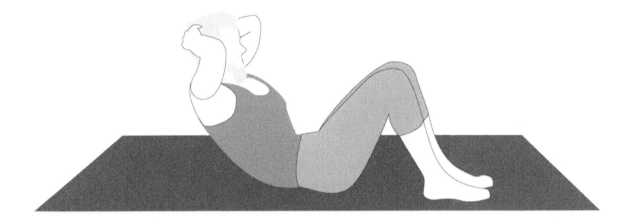

One of the most important core exercises is the crunch.

This exercise is usually combined with lifting the legs and arms with the abdomen resting on the mat. The extension of the muscle bands makes it possible to significantly reduce back pain, improve the core and strengthen the abdomen.

Lie on the ground on your back and with the soles of your feet flat on the floor, hip-width apart.

Bend your knees and place your arms crossed on your chest.

Contract your abs and inhale. Exhale and raise your upper body, keeping your head and neck relaxed, avoiding bending your back.

Raising your pelvis while lying on the mat also significantly helps your back, offering immediate relief when done with correct timing and without quick jerking.

FRONT PLANK

With your forearms resting on the ground under your body from the prone position, lift your hips and torso off the floor, making sure to keep you arms straight.

The body must remain aligned from the ankles to the neck, with the back and hips as straight as possible.

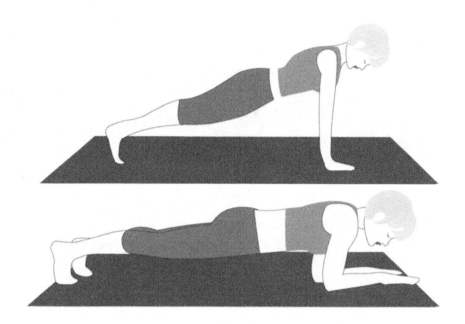

It is an isometric exercise that can also be performed in repetitions.

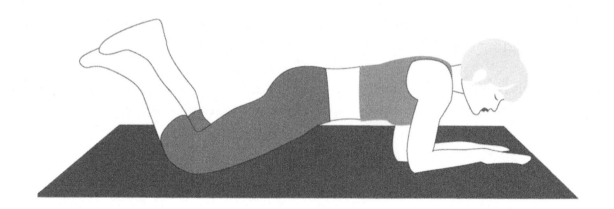

PLANK LEG LIFTS

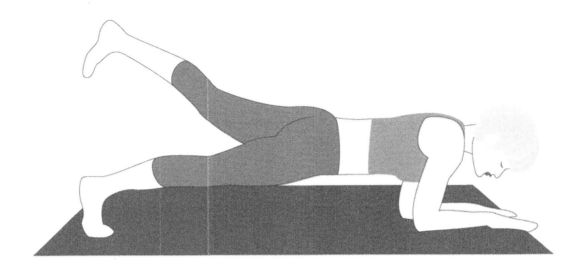

It is a variant of the previous one that also stimulates the gluteus maximus.

It simply involves alternating leg swings backward, taking the feet off the floor.

This too can be done in isometry or alternating.

You can try the variant on the forearms if the engagement is painful or uncomfortable.

Chapter 10
Weight Exercises

Social isolation is a complex challenge; after the Covid experience, we know that for sure. Still, there is absolutely some work we can do to improve exercise at home.

Over the years, a sort of fragility arises in the body, accompanied by an involuntary weight loss, a slower walk, widespread muscle weakness, and fatigue, leading to lower levels of activity that do nothing but make things worse.

Maintaining and building core muscle strength, we have repeated this several times, is the key.

Well: weight training, which perhaps progresses with intensity, is very effective in countering the decline in health with aging.

A research published by the Journal of Frailty and Aging measured the muscle strength and performance levels of a group of seniors who had consistently trained their core for 12 weeks compared to those who didn't. The first group had improved their muscle performance, walking speed, grip strength, and time to stand up while seated. Many of these changes were already visible after nine weeks.

Traditionally, older adults opt for low-intensity, low-resistance exercises because they believe heavy activity is not suitable for them. The results of this study demonstrated the opposite.

Before training with weights, however, here are some rules to follow for proper execution:

- priority to the correct posture of the exercises over the loads;
- education in load progression;
- controlled and pain-free movement;
- avoid blocking breathing;
- pay attention to the eccentric phases of the movements;
- never exceed the training hour.

EXERCISES FOR BEGINNERS

Get a pair of 2 kg dumbbells or two full one-and-a-half-liter bottles of water. Get the mat, choose a safe environment... and start!

As we said before your workout (and before EVERY workout), do at least 5 minutes of warm-up.

CURL WITH WEIGHTS

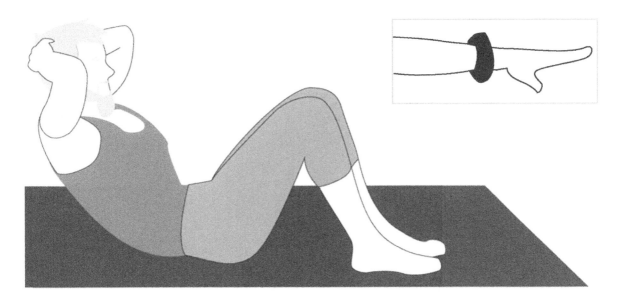

Position yourself with your arms on the ground, perpendicular to the ground, and hold the dumbbells with the classic neutral grip (neutral grip = palms facing inwards).

Begin the movement by flexing the elbow while moving the arms.

Flex the humerus slightly and then return to the starting position.

Remember to keep your elbow firmly attached to your torso when doing this workout and make quiet movements without overdoing it.

Furthermore, it is essential to maintain the right concentration throughout the workout to avoid any kind of error.

STRAIGHT-LEG DETACHMENTS

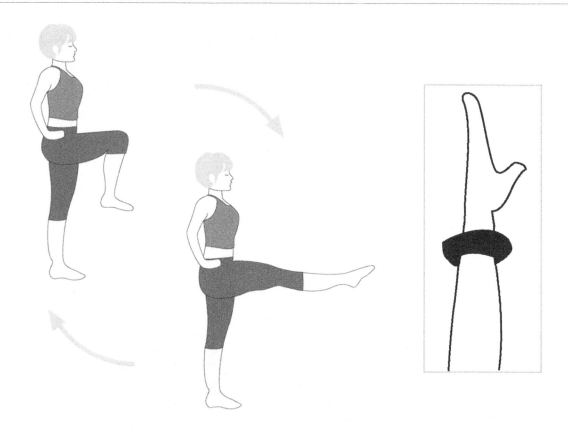

In this exercise, the legs are practically stiff as you perform it.

In the case of a normal deadlift, the knees bend much more.

If you find it hard to lean forward without hunching your back, work on the flexibility of your hamstrings.

You can freely replace the exercise with a normal deadlift by adding weights.

Special attention to the shape:
- Contract your abs and back;
- It is okay to maintain a neutral arch with the back,. It is not good if the back curves in the other direction (flexing the spine);
- Start the movement by pushing your hips back;
- Bend your knees as necessary to avoid hunching your back (hamstring flexibility can limit movement).

OARSMAN FOLDED FORWARD

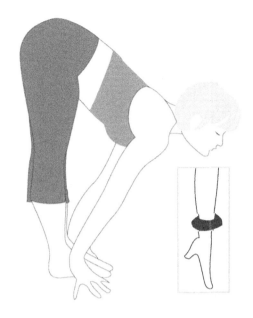

Start from the standing position, grab the dumbbells, and, keeping your back straight, bend forward until you reach an angle of 45 °.

Activates the shoulder blades and the core, pushing the buttocks outwards by slightly bending the legs downwards and with a soft wrist.

Then go down with the weights towards the floor, then rise again, bringing them towards the navel. The elbows remain close to the body.

Do all repetitions with one arm, then switch sides.

EXERCISES FOR ADVANCED

ONE-LEGGED DEADLIFT

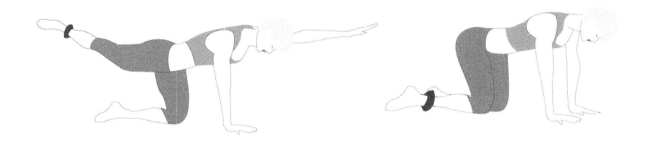

In the quadrupedal position, on the hands and mat, with the back parallel to the floor, extend one arm forward taking the dumbbells and the contralateral leg back, pointing outward.

It is an exercise that can be done in isometry or alternating repetitions on both sides.

Make sure not to lower your hips and shoulders and arch your back.

SQUAT BICYCLE CRUNCH

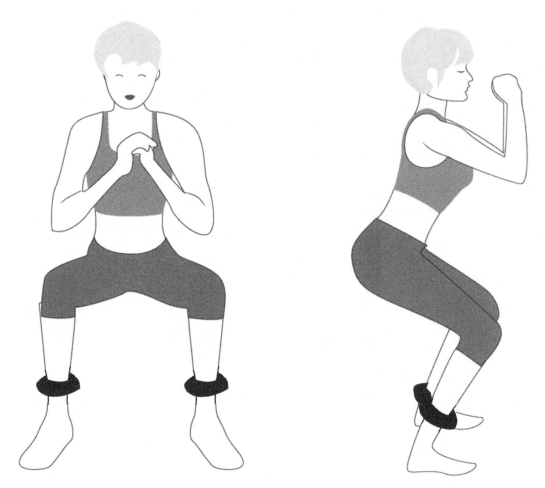

Start   in a
standing position, with feet hip-width apart, elbows high, fingertips close to the temples,
and palms facing outwards.

Go down into a squat, then stand up and bring the left knee up and to the right,
simultaneously moving the right elbow down and to the left so that the left knee and the
right elbow come together.

Return to the starting position, descend into a squat, then rotate and perform a crunch on
the opposite side.

Continue the same sequence, alternating sides.

LUNGES IN MOTION

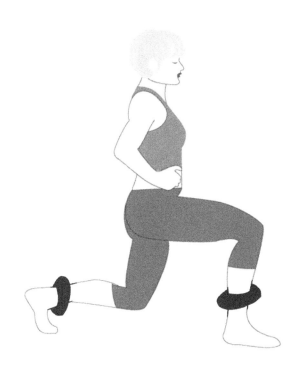

Start with your feet hip-distance apart and your hands on your hips.

Perform a lunge by stepping forward with the left foot, bringing the left knee in line with the left forefoot and the right knee lightly touching the floor.

Then, applying pressure through your left foot, step forward with your right foot. Repeat on the right side.

If it is too difficult, make reverse lunges while standing, or make standing lunges and place a pillow under your knees.

If it's too easy, make walking lunges with a weight plate above your head.

SIDE LUNGES

Start from a standing position. Your feet are hip-width apart.

In one smooth motion, lift the right foot and, keeping the left foot straight, spread the right foot, coming down into a squat on the right leg, keeping the knee in line with the right forefoot, with the hands slightly together and in front of the body as a counterweight.

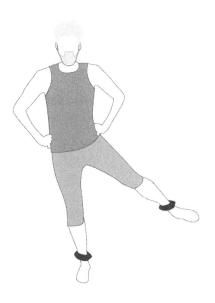

Return to your starting position. Repeat on the left side.

Chapter 11
Strength and Aerobic Exercises

Motor training must be personalized, so each elderly person can have different problems, which must be kept in mind to avoid worsening the situation.

For example, letting an elderly person who shows some balance difficulties practice cycling - however quietly - would greatly increase the risk of a fall and bone fracture. As we know, rupture of the femur is one of the main causes of bed rest and even death in old age. And so on.

Furthermore, in arthritic people, especially inoperable ones, the active mobilization of the affected district is not always an appropriate choice; putting too much strain on an already painful joint can lead to worsening painful symptoms and consequent reduction of mobility.

Overall, physical activity for seniors must engage both aerobic metabolism - which has an excellent impact on blood parameters, and respiratory and cardio-circulatory fitness - and the expression of strength, maintaining muscle tropism.

Aerobic exercises

Aerobic activities for seniors should be low intensity and medium volume. It means that the heartbeat, as well as the respiratory rate, should not indicate an excess of breathlessness. The total duration could be 20-30 seconds.

The daily movement offers the best results, but if this is not possible, it is advisable to stick to 3-4 sessions per week. But don't worry: all kinds of movements are fine.

For those who have the opportunity, even with a cane or walker, walking is welcome. The same applies to bicycle use. On the other hand, if it is not possible outdoors, we recommend using a treadmill or exercise bike - always useful.

6 STRENGTHENING EXERCISES (WITH BANDS)

As for the musculation, we will now make a few examples that should cover most of the catchment area in old age. Even in this case, the optimal frequency would be daily, given the modest time commitment they occupy. Still, 3-4 times a week is perfectly fine. All you need is a rubber band and a chair.

One last thing: it is advisable to have the exercises illustrated by an expert, especially if it's the first time.

UP AND DOWN FROM THE CHAIR

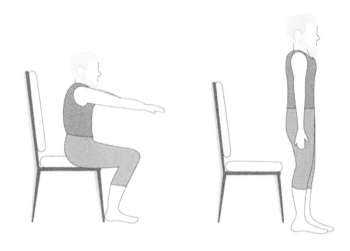

With the help of a table, place your hands on a table (typical meal position): to be done calmly about 20 times.

STANDING TWIST

Standing, rotate the torso from side to side, keeping the legs still shoulder-width apart. Repeat it for about 30 seconds.

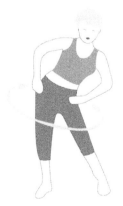
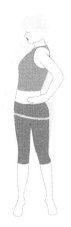

BENDING FORWARD

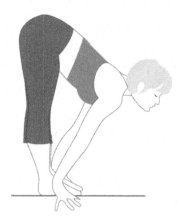

Start from a standing position. Keep your back straight and legs apart, then bend forward as far as possible.

Return to an upright position, vertebra after vertebra. Repeat it about 10-20 times.

ARMS SIDEWAYS

Start from a standing position. Then raise the arms stretched sideways to above the head or as far as the joints allow you to do it. Repeat it about 10-20 times;

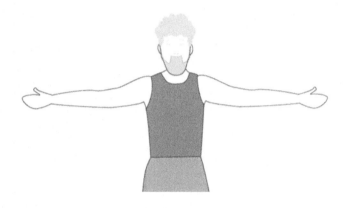

CAT & COW

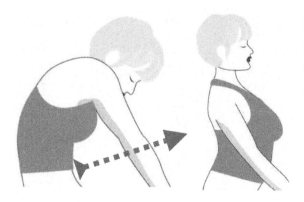

Start from a standing position. Pur your arms extended in front of the torso, then open and close repeatedly but slowly: about 10-20 times.

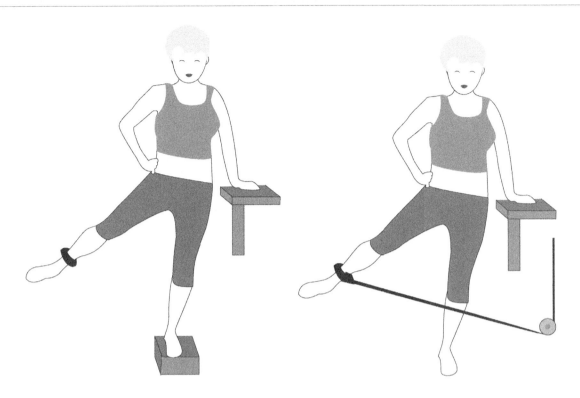

Fix a rubber band to the handle of a door or on the top of a radiator. Then hold it with one outstretched arm at a time.

Push down sideways 10-20 times.

Variant: Use the elastic tied as in the previous exercise above. Hold it from the front, then pull it towards you. Make sure to flex the elbow and hold it close to the side, about 10-20 times.

Chapter 12
Cooling Down

The cooldown, or cool down, goes hand in hand with the warm-up or warm-up. While the warm-up phase prepares your muscles for physical activity, the cooldown phase helps your body return to its original pre-workout state.

The cooldown allows you to gradually reduce your body temperature. Regular recovery exercises allow for better long-term results and reduce the risk of injury.

The cooldown performs many important functions for your body and muscles:
• Supports and accelerates regeneration;
• Normalizes breathing and the cardiovascular system;
• Speeds up the elimination of metabolites (end products of metabolism), such as lactate;
• It relaxes the muscles and reduces tension;
• Relieves muscle aches;
• Helps to relax the mind.

Here's how you can cool down your core after training.

Cardio

After training, dedicate 10 minutes of cardio at will (a nice walk outside or inside the house is enough).

Choose a moderate pace: the goal is to catch your breath. If you can chat while doing the exercise, it means that the speed is the right one;)

Light cardio activities allow the body to regulate the cardiovascular system and breathing. The metabolites that are formed due to physical activity are eliminated more easily. The recovery time is shortened, and you can give it your all in the next workout.

It is a type of cool down and is particularly suitable after intensive and tiring sessions.

Stretching

Post-activity stretching and stretching exercises (and not before!) can reduce muscle tension and improve blood circulation, which speeds up the elimination of metabolites.

Avoid doing fast dynamic stretches because, with sudden movements, you will get the opposite effect to the desired one. The muscles would find themselves in an alternating state between tension and relaxation and would not be able to relax.

Hot shower

After training, you can also choose to take a hot shower (or a sauna). Heat expands blood vessels, improves circulation, and promotes regeneration.

Body and mind relax and regain energy. In addition, heat can have a positive effect on sore muscles and accelerate regeneration.

Give your body a short break before taking a shower to slow blood circulation. Also, ensure you have drunk enough and if the heat is right for your body condition (ask your doctor for advice).

Massages

Massages are ideal in the cooldown phase. The fasciae and muscles loosen, and the tension decreases. This causes muscle pains to be reduced.

Try to apply light and gentle pressure to avoid counterproductive muscle effects.

6 COOL-DOWN EXERCISES AFTER WORKOUT

1

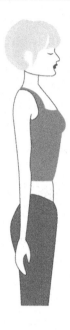

Feet parallel slightly apart so that they are at shoulder height, heels fixed on the ground, legs bent, and torso in a semi-sitting position, ensuring that the back remains straight.

By assuming this position, the quadriceps (front of the thigh) will be in tension, but the rear muscles will be able to relax;

2

Standing with one hand against the wall, bring the heel of one leg to the buttock and grab the foot or ankle with the hand of the opposite arm.

Gently pull while maintaining the axis of the back, pelvis, and legs. This stretches the quadriceps.

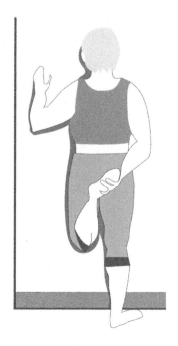

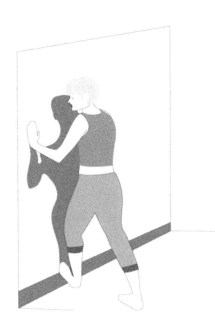

 To tension the Achilles tendon, place your arms on a wall or chair and flex the leg that is left behind by lowering the pelvis.

5. Use the bench or a chair to place one foot on it so that the leg is raised and the knee is bent sufficiently.

The foot on the ground should be straight with the heel resting on the floor; the other leg should almost be stretched back.

Push your pelvis forward until you feel the tension in your thigh and groin.

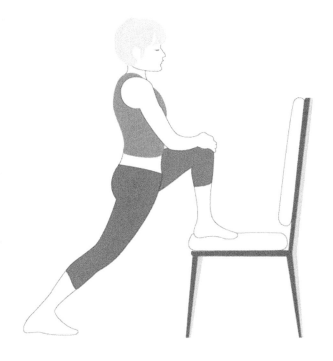

5

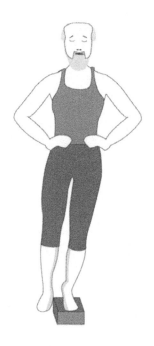
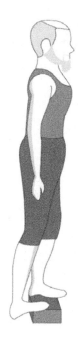

Lift one leg sideways and place it on a support, and keep the other foot with the heel fixed on the ground with the toe straight forward.

Reached the position, slowly approached the shoulder to the raised knee, making a bow and slightly rotating the pelvis inwards.

This stretches the adductor muscles in the leg.

6

Leaning on the palms of the hands and knees, assuming the position of the dog upside down and slightly arching the back: an ideal position to stretch the whole body.

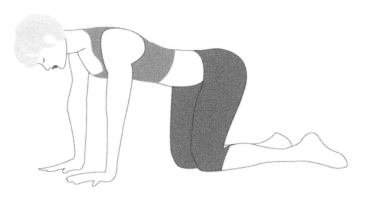

It is good to remember that they vary according to the type of activity performed and the muscles involved in the workout.

It is good to rely on the advice of an expert who can guide you in choosing the exercises that best suit your case.

Chapter 13
Weekly Schedules

You may ask yourself: how can I integrate these core and strength exercises into my daily routine? We have also thought about this!

Take these tips as such: always ask a specialist or your doctor for advice first.
Also, determine how many times you want to train your strength, in conjunction with everything you can do regarding training.

The ideal would be at least three times a week, but then again: it's up to you!
Here is an ideal weekly routine for core and strength training:

Monday	Tuesday	Wednesday	Thursday	Friday	Saturday	Sunday
Seated	Standing	Mat	*Rest*	Seated	Standing	Mat

SEATED FLOW: MONDAY / FRIDAY

FORWARD FOLD

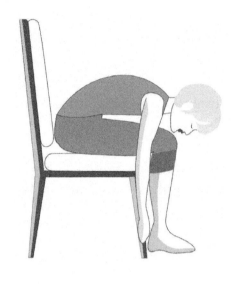

Inhale and raise your arms.

Then as you exhale, lean forward, resting your torso on your thighs.

If possible, place your hands on the floor and dangle your head. Rest in this position for a few breaths.

To exit, straighten your arms in front of you above your head and come up.

Repeat three times in total, and the last time you bend forward, stay there.

RECLINED CURL

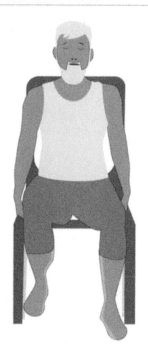

Sit on a chair, placing your feet firmly on the ground and contracting your core muscles and abdominals for at least one minute.

Keep the spine straight while inhaling and bringing the head back.

Stop just before touching the backrest, exhaling as you return to the starting position.

Perform two sets of five repetitions each.

SIDE BENDS

Start in a sitting position, with your back resting on the back of the chair, your legs touching, and your feet firmly planted on the ground.

Slowly raise one hand and put it on the same side knee. Then bend your torso on the opposite side, arms straight, punting on the floor, trying to touch the floor with your fingertips.

Hold the position for 3-4 inhalation and exhalation cycles.Repeat on the second side.

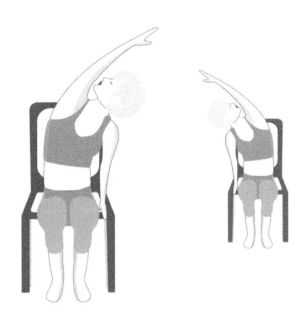

SHOULDER ROUNDS

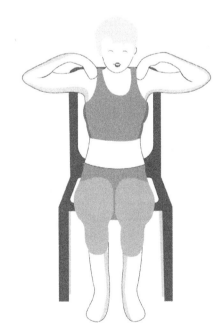

Moving the shoulders is essential to promote mobility and warm up the body before the practice.

Sit straight with your chest open and your feet firmly on the floor.

Then slowly, move your shoulders up and down, back and forth, and then proceed with backward rotations.

Breathing from the abdomen with each movement is vital to relax the muscles and prepare us for our practice.

You can use slow exhalations, counting 4 to inhale and 8 to exhale. Gradually increase the number of exhalations to 12 and 16. This system has an immediate calming effect on the nervous system.

CACTUS

A simple position but capable of giving tone, strength, and energy to the body and arms.

Start in a sitting position, with your back resting on the back of the chair, your legs touching, and your feet firmly planted on the ground.

Then slowly raise your arms by bending your elbows to form a right angle with your body, to look a bit like a giant cactus.

Stretching your stomach in, lean forward slowly, remembering to breathe. Then, vertebra after vertebra, pull yourself up and repeat the exercise 10 times.

Then lower your arms.

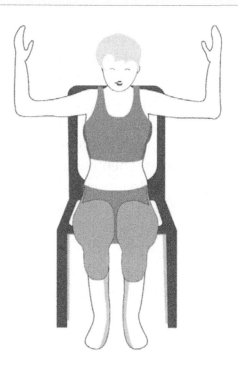

SCISSORS

Sitting on the edge of the chair, firmly grasp the sides of the chair with both legs.

Then proceed by extending your legs with the toes pointing upwards, trying to keep your back straight.

Inhale and pull your belly in, then begin to slowly lift your legs, alternating them as high as possible, before slowly returning to the starting position.

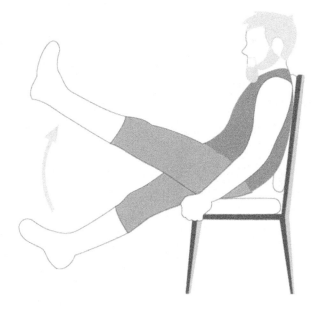

SQUEEZING THE KNEES

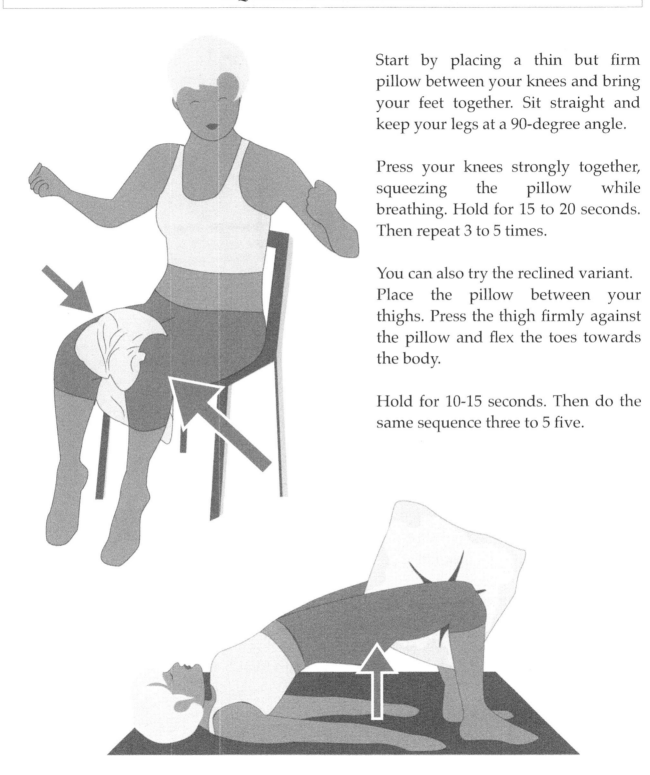

Start by placing a thin but firm pillow between your knees and bring your feet together. Sit straight and keep your legs at a 90-degree angle.

Press your knees strongly together, squeezing the pillow while breathing. Hold for 15 to 20 seconds. Then repeat 3 to 5 times.

You can also try the reclined variant. Place the pillow between your thighs. Press the thigh firmly against the pillow and flex the toes towards the body.

Hold for 10-15 seconds. Then do the same sequence three to 5 five.

BOAT POSE

Start by sitting in the mat chair with your knees facing forward and your feet flat on the floor.

Move to the edge of the chair; lean back slightly, and place your hands behind you on the chair.

As you exhale, lift your feet off the floor and bring your knees towards your chest. During the entire process, keep your back straight and engage your abdominal muscles

If you find this posture simple, you can also add balance to the pose by lifting your arms close to your legs.

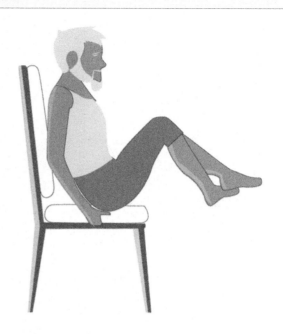

Continue to breathe deeply while holding this position for 30 seconds to one minute. To release, slowly lower your feet to the floor and sit straight.

Repeat two or three times, never forgetting to breathe deeply!

REST PEACEFULLY

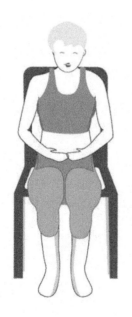

To perform this pose, stand still with your feet planted on the ground.

And then put your hands on your stomach, inserting inhalations and exhalations of equal length.

Closes your eyes and breath for 4-5 cycles of inhale/exhale.

NECK AND SHOULDERS RELEASE

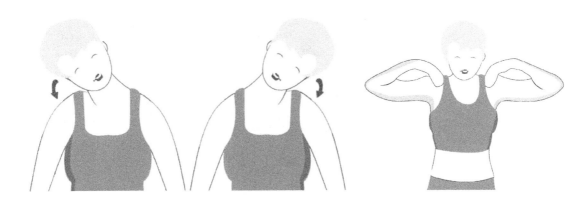

Starts by standing, with your shoulders down, your neck muscles relaxed, and hands on your knees.

You will need to move your head in coordination with your breath.

Look up and go back to the center; look down and go back to the center. Then look towards the right and left shoulder and finally bring your ear to one shoulder and the other.

Close the pose with a neck circle, first clockwise and then counterclockwise.

Move slowly, slower than you would, and open your eyes to prevent dizziness.

Then, move your shoulders up and down, back and forth, and then proceed with backward rotations.

Breathing from the abdomen with each movement is vital to relax the muscles and prepare us for our practice.

You can use slow exhalations, counting 4 to inhale and 8 to exhale. Gradually increase the number of exhalations to 12 and 16. This system has an immediate calming effect on the nervous system.

HIPS CIRCLES

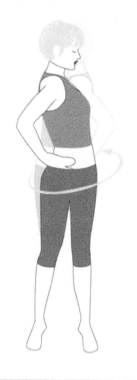
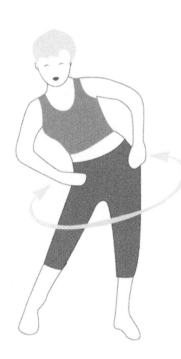

Stand with your legs slightly apart; put your hands on your hips. Make circular movements clockwise for thirty seconds. Now, for another thirty seconds, perform the same movements counterclockwise.

HALF SQUATS

Stand upright, with legs apart, feet turned slightly outward, and hands resting on thighs. You can use a wall behind you if it's more comfortable. Then bend the knees while keeping your back straight.

Stop before the buttocks reach the level of the knees.

Exhale and return to the starting position.

Perform three sets of ten repetitions each.

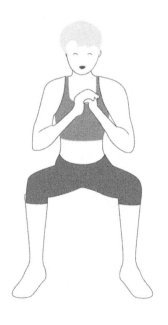
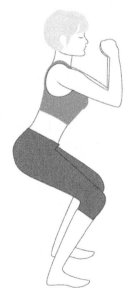

Standing erect with feet together and hands on hips.

As you lift your left leg to the side, exhale and return to the starting position.

Keep the trunk and shoulders aligned throughout the movement by contracting the abdomen. Maintain unaltered curves of the spine. Stabilize the supporting leg by contracting the buttocks and abdomen.

Perform all repetitions, then repeat with the right leg.

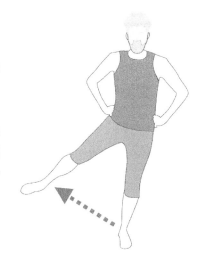

FRONT LEGS RAISE

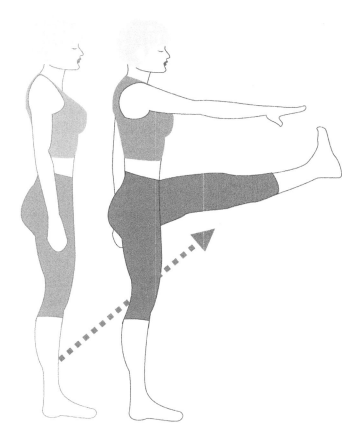

Start from a standing position. Keep both feet on the ground and arms at your sides for balance.

Lift the right knee upwards as far as possible, then lower the foot to the ground.
Maintain unaltered curves of the spine.

Stabilize the supporting leg by contracting the buttocks and abdomen.

Perform all repetitions, then repeat with the left leg.

HALF LUNGES

Stand upright, keeping your feet together and your arms at your sides.

Step forward and bend your left leg to form a right angle.

From the starting position, repeat the same movement on the other side.

Distribute your body weight evenly between the right and left foot. The back, shoulder, hip, and knee should be aligned in the lunge position.

Do three sets of ten repetitions each.

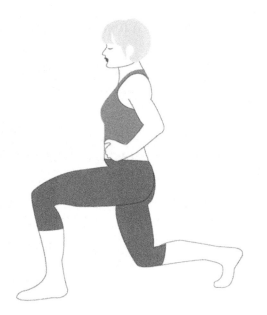

STANDING PUNCH

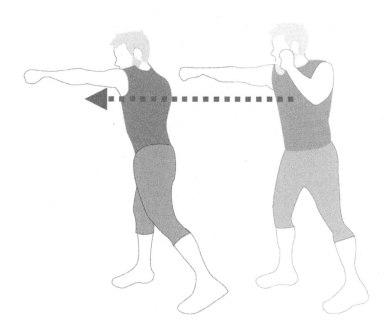

From a standing position, keep your feet shoulder-width apart.

Bring the rib cage in and strengthen the core by pulling the navel towards the spine and keeping the pelvis in traction.

Extend your arms alternately, punching the air imaginary, alternating sides, and gradually increasing the pace.

QUADRICEPS

Hold on to the chair or a wall with your left hand. Bend your right knee.

Grab your leg by the ankle with your right hand and gently pull your foot towards your bottom. Stay in the position for 10 to 20 seconds.

Put your leg back down and repeat with your left leg.

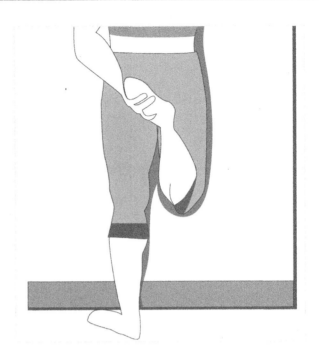

ABDOMINAL VACUUM

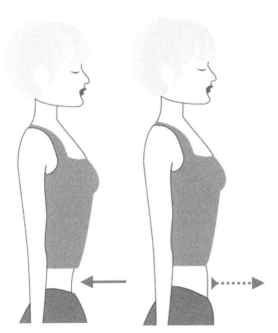

Stand upright with your hands on your hips. Breathe in.

The position is easily performed by the voluntary movement of pushing the belly in and, forcing exhalation, throwing the air out.

BUTTERFLY

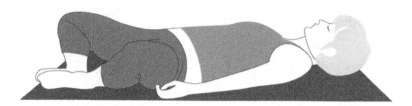

Lay down on the mat, and extend your legs.

Bring the knees out to the side, with the soles of the feet together. Try to make a diamond shape with your legs.

Rest in this pose, staying there for 5 to ten breaths, placing your hands on your belly or out to the sides.

To come out from the pose, roll onto one side and use your hands to help you back up to sitting.

CAT AND COW

Start on all fours, and bring your hands with your shoulders and knees in line with your hips. Your back parallels the floor while contracting the abdomen, pulling the navel towards the spine.

From this position, inhale, open your chest, bring your shoulder blades closer and look up: this is the cow's position.

Then, exhale, make a hump with your back, create space between the shoulder blades, and pull the navel in: this is the cat's position.

Repeat the sequence at least five times.

TWIST

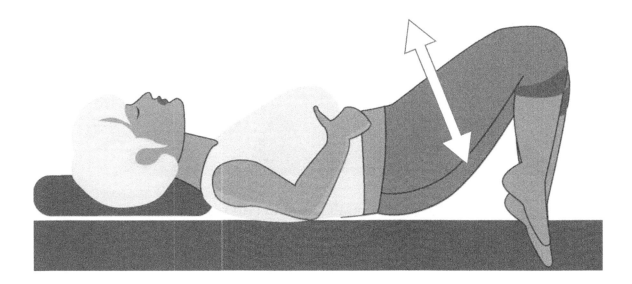

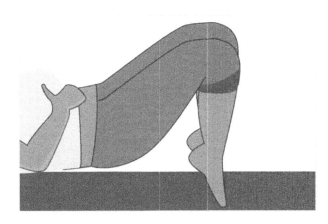

Start by sitting comfortably on the mat, bending the knees.
Then start taking a deep inhalation.

As you exhale, gently rotate your torso to the right, turning your head as well. Place your left hand on your right knee and your right hand on the back of the mat.

Hold this twist for 3-4 breaths. Then gently return to the neutral position.

At this point, do this very same twist on the left side.

Hold this position for 3-4 breaths. Then return to the starting position; proceed to alternate the two rotations for at least 2-3 minutes.

CURL

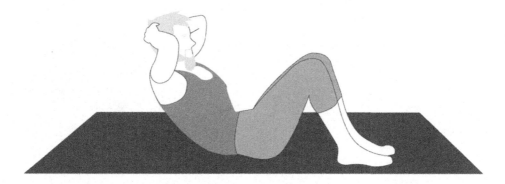

Lie on the mat, placing your feet firmly on the ground and contracting your core muscles and abdominals for at least one minute.

Keep the spine straight while inhaling and bringing the head back.

Exhaling as you return to the starting position.

Perform two sets of five repetitions each, never forgetting to breathe deeply!

CHILD POSE

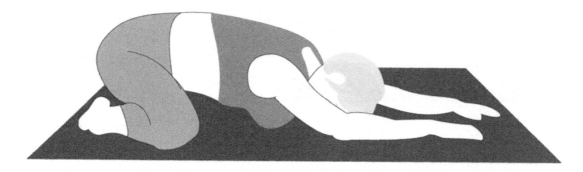

Kneel, bring your big toes against each other, and spread your knees. Bring the torso towards the ground between the thighs, extend the arms in front of you, but relax the neck and shoulders. Bring your forehead to the ground and leave your elbows bent.
With each exhalation, feel how the pelvis relaxes in the direction of the heels. Observe breathing in your back; imagine a balloon inflating and deflating. Maintain for at least one and a half minutes.

BRIDGE

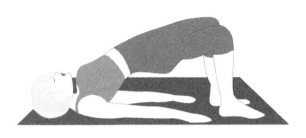

Lie on your back: your arms at your sides and palms facing down.

Then bend your knees, rests your feet on the floor below the knees, and spread your legs to the same width as the hips.

Press your feet to the floor, lift your hips and create a straight line from the knees to the shoulders.

Then squeeze the glute and pulls the navel back towards the spine.

Bring the weight of the body on the shoulder blades and the upper back, do not keep the load of the body resting on the neck.

You can perform the basic bridge statically by holding the position for 20 to 30 seconds, or actively bringing your hips up and down without touching the floor, 15-30 times.

Repeat the exercise for 2-3 laps.

SAVASANA

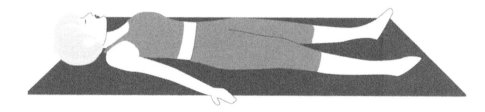

As the name suggests, the Savasana remains perfectly still, in a prone position, with the arms extended along the body and the eyes closed for a sufficient period, not less than 5 minutes, to reach rest, calm and inner peace.

Make sure you don't fall asleep.

BOOK 4:
BALANCE EXERCISES FOR SENIORS FOR FALLING PREVENTION

Chapter 1
Never Falling Again

The relationship between seniors and balance is a very delicate relationship. Falls and unstable balance are among the most common clinical problems after a certain age. They can cause fractures and injuries, which, in a significant percentage of cases, lead to immobilization and are life-threatening.

Just think that according to the American Centers for Disease Control and Prevention, falls are the most common cause of injury in the elderly, with more than one in four elderly falling each year: of these falls, one in five reasons serious injuries such as broken bones or head injury.

According to the World Health Organization (WHO), moreover, 4 out of 10 people aged 65 and over fall every year in the world. 5 out of 10 people over 70. This is why it is essential to act preventively, taking all possible precautions to reduce the risks.

Among the things the elderly can do to protect themselves is specific gymnastics and exercises, that improve balance and stability and lower falls.

And that's exactly why we are here for!

The more years pass, the more the chances of falling and, therefore, of getting traumas increase. For what reasons? We should note that some medications, middle ear problems, and vision loss - all common after a certain age - can affect balance, increasing the likelihood of falling. Even the loss of muscle mass, in some ways inevitable with aging, represents a problem not just: to have specific stability and a good balance, you need to have strong muscles.

Balance and strength routines and exercises, then, are really important and can help prevent falls by improving your ability to control and maintain your body position during movement and when standing still.

Chapter 2
Inner and Outer Balance

The cooldown, or cool down, goes hand in hand with the warm-up or warm-up. While Sometimes I hear clients say: 'You know, I'm wrong to the right (or left), I'm not in balance because I carry my bag …'. I ask them: "Are you in balance? Internal/ Inner and External/ Outer?'

Human being is a perfect machine, a set of its components: physical, emotional, and spiritual ... and do you think we can get twisted for a bag?

I'll give you the example of a man who lives this life: his wife cheats on him, he doesn't talk to his children, he is mistreated at work, friends are just a distant memory, he lives in a house polluted by mold and smokes wildly, he hasn't been physically active for 20 years, and I could go on another five lines to write things that are devastating for his health, and he says: 'You know, I'm wrong to the right (or left) because I carry my bag ..'.

Live a life if you don't belong and blame the bag; that poor thing is the one that makes you feel bad? Let's start looking inside and understanding who we are and how we live before blaming the bag ;)

So how can balance issues affect health?

My first Yoga teacher used to say something that made us students laugh, but over time I fully understood: 'Better to have 20 kg on your shoulders every day than 1 kg of poop in the belly!' The skeleton was made to protect, support, and make us move. Everything inside must work at its best to have health outside, including the intestine.

Do you know that if you are physically centered (therefore without joint or visceral blocks that alter your balance), you are also more emotionally centered, and therefore, you are stronger and more ready to 'face the things you live' or bad luck that happen to you?

Until I was 20, I thought that the inside and the outside of the body were two different things, separate, detached from each other, and I thought it was possible only by eating one thing or another or taking medicine. I would also have changed the outside of my body… and the first times I studied or told the opposite, I was very skeptical.

Now, after 20 years of studying, researching, and applying what I have learned, I don't know how I used to live so disconnected from the internal 'me' and the reality of the body and life!

That's the whole point of this chapter: the internal balance equals the external balance (in all its forms!)

Many times it happens to me that after a series of sessions, people tell me that they have experienced changes, not only postural or pain, but are stronger in certain situations and circumstances from which they previously could not come out ... even in the field of relationships, personal or business. When people realize these things in a very short time, it is a real and profound joy for me!

I have thrown many seeds into your vegetable garden called the brain, and I hope they grow and become colorful and fragrant flowers and make you understand that we are not a bunch of bones, ligaments, and tendons but we are much, much more!

The same Yogi who explained the poop in the belly of the above example told us: 'Don't get mad like dogs on the bone!' Bone is a fundamental part of the body, but it is not the only one; on the contrary ... it works with everything else, fully integrated into the 'human system' and regulates its functions in every small part.

I'm talking to you about something that you certainly consider fundamental for the health of your body: blood. Do you know that it is closely related to bone functioning? Yes, you got it right. If our skeleton (bone) is functioning well, the production of red blood cells, platelets, and most of the leukocytes (white blood cells) are also produced correctly! Bone marrow (red) is found mainly in flat bones such as the skull, vertebrae, shoulder blades and the spongy tissue of the long bones (femur and humerus) and produces these blood elements. Are you shocked by this link? Sometimes when a person says to me: "I did a sprain, but it won't affect the rest of my body, will it?" I start talking and never finish explaining the problems this ankle will bring if not treated properly!

This example of the correlation between bone and blood is just an example of how much we are connected and how important the inside is with the outside.

Working, therefore, for the construction of an external balance, even and above all as the elderly, becomes essential to rediscover that inner dedication, that well-being, and that love for ourselves that we have waxed throughout our life. In one word: balance! And it's never too late to find it!

Chapter 3
Fall Risk Factors

With 'balance disorder' in medicine, we mean a condition that makes the individual who suffers from it perceive a sense of dizziness or instability in posture as if he were in motion while standing upright or lying down.

These disorders can be caused by certain health conditions, drugs, or a problem with the inner ear or brain. The medical term used to identify all parts of the inner ear involved in the balance mechanism is the vestibular system. It controls the sense of balance, posture, body orientation in space, locomotion, and other movements. In addition, it helps preserve objects' focus when the body is in motion.

The vestibular system works concurrently with other sensory systems in the body (for example, eyes, bones, and joints) to control and maintain the body's position at rest and in motion.

The sense of balance, moreover, is mainly controlled by a labyrinthine structure in the inner ear called the labyrinth. The semicircular canals and the otolithic organs present within the labyrinth helps to maintain balance.

Balance disorder: what are the symptoms?

Symptoms can appear and disappear for short periods, or they can last for long periods. Common symptoms of a balance disorder include:
- dizziness or vertigo;
- feeling like you are about to fall;
- lightheadedness, fainting, or a sensation of floating;
- blurred vision;
- confusion or disorientation;
- nausea and vomit;
- diarrhea;
- changes in blood pressure and heart rate;
- fear;

- anxiety;
- panic.

What can be the causes of a balance disorder?

A balance disorder can be caused by bacterial or viral ear infections, head injuries, or blood circulation disorders affecting the inner ear or brain.

Many people experience problems with the sense of balance as they age. Problems with balance and dizziness can also be caused by taking some medications. The issues affecting the nervous and circulatory systems can be the source of some difficulties with posture and balance.

Issues related to skeletal or visual systems, such as arthritis or imbalance of the ocular muscles, can also cause balance problems.

However, many balance disorders can start suddenly without any apparent cause.

These are some possible causes of loss of balance (it is not an exhaustive list; it's always better to consult your doctor if symptoms persist):

- Alcoholism;
- Brain aneurysm;
- Transient ischemic attack;
- Motion sickness;
- Cholecystitis;
- Vascular dementia;
- Dyspraxia;
- Sprained Ankle;
- Cerebral hemorrhage;
- Wernicke's encephalopathy;
- Stroke;
- Influence;
- Carbon monoxide poisoning;
- Cerebral ischemia;
- Labyrinthitis;
- Acoustic neuroma;
- Neurofibromatosis;
- Vestibular neuronitis;
- Ear infection;
- Barotraumatic otitis;
- Otosclerosis;

- Hollow foot;
- Flatfoot;
- Amyotrophic lateral sclerosis;
- Decompression syndrome;
- Fibromyalgia syndrome;
- Essential thrombocythemia.

How is a balance disorder diagnosed?

Diagnosing a balance disorder is difficult. There are many potential causes, including medical conditions and medications. To facilitate the assessment of the problem, the doctor may suggest that the patient refers to an otolaryngologist (doctor and surgeon specializing in the ears, nose, and throat).

The otolaryngologist can recommend a hearing test, blood tests, and electronystagmography (an examination that analyzes eye movements and the muscles that control them) tests with images to study the head and brain.

Another possible exam is called posturography. The patient must stand on a unique mobile platform before a screen. Using this test, the physician evaluates how the patient's body moves in response to the movement of the platform, the screen, or both.

How is it treated?

A doctor's first assessment is to determine whether the patient's dizziness is caused by a medical condition or by taking medications. If these factors are found, the doctor will treat the disease or suggest a different medication to the patient.

The treatment for the balance disorders described above will depend on the specific balance disorder.

Some other treatment options include taking medications, vestibular rehabilitation therapy, exercises for the head, body, and eyes, and modifications to household appliances to make the home safer (for example, the installation of handrails at home).

What are the remedies for the loss of balance?

Sometimes the loss of balance is a momentary disturbance. Other times it is necessary to act on the health problem that triggers the disorder. This is why it is essential to consult a doctor. I t may be required to change the intake of some medications, or changes in diet, physiotherapy, or exercises to be performed at home may be helpful to reduce the risk of getting hurt. Other times it is necessary to solve the problem by taking medications (for example, antibiotics against infection, nausea, or corticosteroids for dizziness). Finally, it may be necessary to intervene surgically, for example, if you suffer from Ménière's syndrome.

When to contact your doctor

In case of loss of balance, it is good to contact your doctor to identify the cause of the problem and deal with it most appropriately. If it is suspected that the problem may be associated with a stroke, it is essential to call an ambulance immediately.

What can you do about it?

Although, as we have seen in the previous pages, falls and balance problems can arise from more severe pathologies, which must be excluded, there is a good chance that they are only a normal part of the aging process. Which, however, you can help slow down or stop altogether. How? I'll explain it to you with the exercises in the following chapters!

Chapter 4
Your Health at Stake

Notwithstanding the physical risks for the elderly, the lack of balance and the fear of falling bring worry and insecurity. Falls threaten independence and self-esteem, especially if they recur, and undermine confidence in leaving the house by accelerating the appearance of:
- the decline of their functions;
- depression;
- social isolation.

You often do not want to tell it, especially to family members and the general practitioner, out of shame or fear of being limited in activities. Still, that's exactly the first step to take.

The physical implications of a fall

The main physical consequence of an accidental fall is a reduction in daily life activities and, therefore, in movement.

I state that advancing age, in addition to wisdom, brings with it other less pleasant aspects related to regular physiological changes:
- Reduction of protective reflexes: you know when you take a retort for a hole, but are you able to regain your balance without even knowing how? It is a reflex that you do not voluntarily check;
- Reduced coordination,
- The appearance of muscle weakness is caused mostly by other pathologies and not moving enough;
- Alterations in balance include the need for support while walking or on the stairs, standing with your legs apart if you are standing, and skidding while walking;
- Stiffness and limitation of movement: do you feel stiff or unable to move as in the past? It could be mainly due to arthrosis; click here to learn more;

- Alteration of the quality of the walk: do you scrape your feet on the ground? Is your stride shorter, or are you walking slower? Do you feel all bent over?
- Osteopenia (the bone becomes thinner and less robust), sarcopenia (the muscle loses some of its mass and strength), osteoporosis (the bone becomes more fragile and more at risk of fracture);
- Increased tissue healing time (think fracture or wound, for example);
- Reduction of vision or hearing;
- Other concomitant pathologies depend on the person.

Moving less, moreover, worsens these aspects and increases the risk of falling.

So, it is more challenging to adopt quick strategies to prevent falls, and if you fall, there is a greater risk of causing damage. So, can falls be prevented in older people? YES. The first step is knowledge!

Chapter 5
How to Prevent Falling?

Although we'll get to the juicy part of the book shortly, the simple, daily, and powerful exercises you can do to train your balance, here are some tips to avoid falls in the first place. What can you do right away? Maybe you already follow many tricks; try to take a look at the others. The following are the seven most important.

1. Get up gradually and slowly from the bed, chair, or sofa - getting up quickly may cause dizziness;
2. Remember to go to the bathroom before going to bed: you will reduce the possibility of waking up in the middle of the night. If this happens, remember the first rules: get up slowly, put on your shoes, put on your glasses, use walking aids and turn on the lights!
3. Always wear safe shoes, preferably closed at the back and with a non-slippery sole, and comfortable clothing which does not crawl on the ground;
4. Always wear glasses for vision problems and hearing aids, and check for proper function;
5. Always and correctly use aids such as a cane, a walker, or a wheelchair, for example, to walk: no matter whether you have to travel 100 meters or a meter, always move safely;
6. If you use the wheelchair, set it up as close as possible and brake it;
7. Always and correctly use aids such as a cane, a walker, or a wheelchair, for example, to walk: no matter whether you have to travel 100 meters or a meter, always move safely.

Safe at Home

Our home may seem like the safest place to stay, but in reality, 6 out of 10 falls happen at home. Some precautions can limit the risk of falls:

• Do not sit on sofas, chairs or toilets that are too low. The lower the seat, the harder to get up. For the chairs and sofas, you can use cushions under your seat, while for the toilet, there are toilet lifts available in orthopedic stores. If you are outdoors, lean on something stable, or do not hesitate to ask for help if needed, there is nothing wrong;

- Pay extreme attention to children and any pets in the wild, or that the leash does not go around the legs;
- Make sure to have handrails installed on both sides of all stairs;
- Check if there is good lighting (and light switches) at the stairs' top and bottom and the corridors' ends. Keep the night lights in the bedroom and bathroom;
- Do not leave books, papers, clothes, or shoes on the floors or stairs, increasing the risk of tripping and falling;
- Beware of wet or slippery floors and always warn those in the house if a floor is wet or leave a visible clue to warn it. Use products such as waxes sparingly. Outdoors, look carefully at the floors;
- To shower safely, you can use child seats or non-slip mats;
- Remember to go to the bathroom regularly - avoid holding her back and reaching the limit so you don't have to get up quickly or run to the bathroom. If, for various reasons, you are not in reasonable control, try to go to the toilet several times safely;
- Do not use rugs or carpets unless they are firmly fixed to the floor with non-slip strips;
- Place the grab bars near the toilets inside and outside the tub and shower;
- Do not use a stool to pick up items or food placed too high;
- Beware of cats and dogs in the house.

Safe Outside

- Be careful or avoid rough terrain outdoors: always pay attention to the presence of obstacles, steps, or sidewalks that are too high. Watch out for holes or grassy ground that can hide dips or be slippery;
- Beware of crowded places: people are in a hurry, they look at their phones, they are distracted, and the possibility of colliding or being hit is high;
- Always use walking aids if you need them;
- Do not forget what you have already learned in the home tips.

Your Mindful Routines

Even before starting exercising, what can you do right away? Maybe you already follow many tricks; try to take a look at the others.

Before taking action, therefore, here are some valuable tips for setting up a conscious and present routine every day of your life.

And the most exciting aspect is that you don't have to sit still! Getting older, slowing down, and being 'senior' does not mean being afraid of 'breaking down,' avoiding risks ...

in this way, we are only preventing ourselves from continuing to live our best years, that is, those ahead of us!

Quite the opposite is true: becoming aware means accepting who we are, where, and above all 'when' we are, and behaving accordingly to prevent problems. And you can do it safely, but without giving up the fun and joy, that life can offer.

Therefore, it is a priority to encourage movement in all its forms: sitting, lying down, standing, or walking inside and outside the home! It is essential not to sit still for long and to stay active.

Of course, the methods depend on each person's state of health and autonomy (I never tire of repeating checking every choice of movement with their doctors) but, regardless of this, there is always a possibility to do so. Just know how!

Before setting up any training program, then, here's how you can start from daily life activities, your conscious and natural routines:

• Get up and sit down;
• Getting out of bed;
• Walk safely;
• Go up and down the stairs.

You can combine exercises to reduce, improve and prevent:

• Muscle weakness and loss of tone;
• Stiffness and limitations of movement;
• Osteopenia, sarcopenia, and osteoporosis;
• The quality of the journey;
• Balance, reflexes, and coordination.

I know it takes desire and a lot of consistency, but now you know all the benefits associated with the movement.

I am sure that you will consider differently the proposal to go for a walk or get up one more time from the chair from now on.

Get regular checkups to monitor your vision, hearing, blood pressure, dizziness, or other conditions.

Trust professionals to evaluate the right aids for you and how to use them correctly.

If you have already made it this far with commitment, you will have a lot of advice to try immediately!

Chapter 6
Challenge Your Balance: 4 Exercises

Muscle weakness is one of the causes of many falls. The leg muscles, especially the calf, hip, and knee, are critical for strength and balance. You can benefit from basic exercises such as walking or swimming, yoga, and cycling.

In general, to promote balance, strengthen the musculature, and prevent you from falling, it is important:

• Strengthen ankles and calves. You can simply do it by sitting on to the back of the chair and then pushing on tiptoe as high as possible;

• Knee curl. Strengthens the buttock and lower back. Cling to the back of a chair and lift one leg behind, then bend the knee and bring the heel towards the butt before returning it to the starting position;

• Leg extension. Strengthen your thighs. Sit on your chair: your back straight and your feet on the ground. Straighten the first leg in front of you as much as possible, then lower it again and repeat on the other side;

• Check the balance: good balance is essential for preventing falls, as it allows you to control and maintain a stable body position. An excellent way to improve balance is to practice Tai Chi or Yoga and Pilates, all disciplines that help build credit, strength, and confidence.

Let's discover the 4 most impactful exercises for fall prevention!

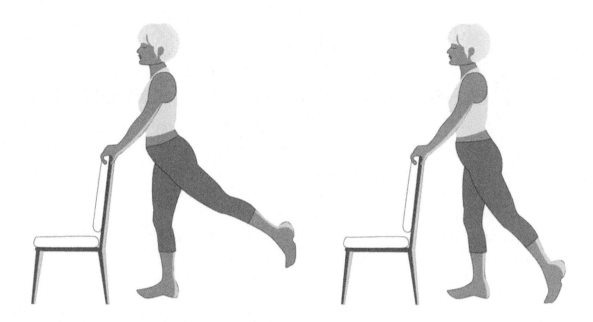

Stand, resting your fingertips on the back of a chair for support.

Lift your right foot off the ground, then slowly rotate it 10 times to the right.

Reverse the direction and rotate the foot 10 more times.

Repeat with the left foot.

As your balance improves, try to stand without support.

EXERCISE 2: STAND AND TAKE A STEP

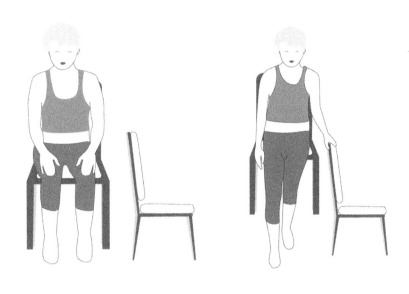

For the first time, you do this just to make sure that you're not gonna lose your balance. This scenario is prevalent. Whether it be to get up, to rush, to go to the bathroom, to answer the phone, to answer the door, it's being able to quickly stand and then shift gears and promptly take that step where the balance problems might occur. So that's again, what we're working on. But in addition to that, I highly recommend that you try doing this without use pushing up from the armrest to add that extra strength challenge to it.

We're gonna start with your feet side by side. And what you're gonna do is just push to standing and immediately go into a step, step it back and down. So you're just gonna try to standing directly, go into a step back, and then down slowly. And then you're gonna switch over to the other leg, using the chair as a support. That's why we have it here.

So this is the central part of this exercise that we're working on is that immediate step that you take right after you stand up out of a chair.

Of course, in an actual situation, you would use the armrest to push up since we're in an exercise mode right now, and we're working on developing strength. If you can try, do try challenging yourself a little bit more by not using the armrest.

And then once you get good at that, and you don't feel like you're gonna lose your balance, you can move both hands to your thighs immediately, go into that step, and then back down.

EXERCISE 3: STEP IN DIFFERENT DIRECTIONS

I love thinking about things like this and creating different situations or different scenarios, or different challenges that will simulate real-life situations. So to change things up a little bit, we don't always step straight ahead. We wanna practice stepping in different directions.

This time, that immediate step is gonna be in a different direction. So you're gonna push and step and back down. So if you need to start, start with your hand right here, push.

So you can see taking that immediate step. And this could really happen in real life when the doorbell rings or when the phone rings.

You're not really thinking, 'I've gotta go sit to stand, gotta make sure I'm balanced. And then I'll take a step.' You're thinking about the phone.

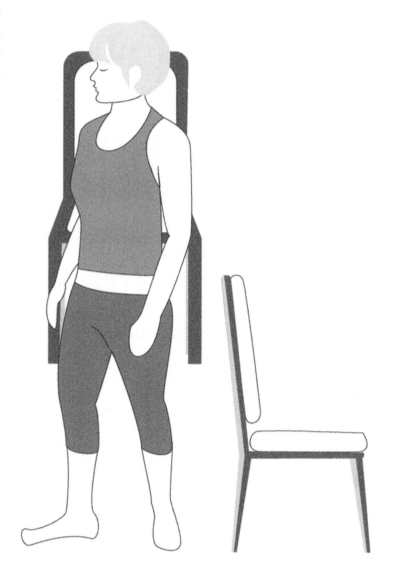

And you're thinking about getting to the bathroom, or you're thinking about the doorbell, and you might not focus as much on standing up, shifting your weight, and taking that step. So practicing.

This will make those reactions more automatic so that you don't need to think about it as much in those scenarios when these situations actually do occur.

EXERCISE 4: PREDICT THE UNPREDICTABLE

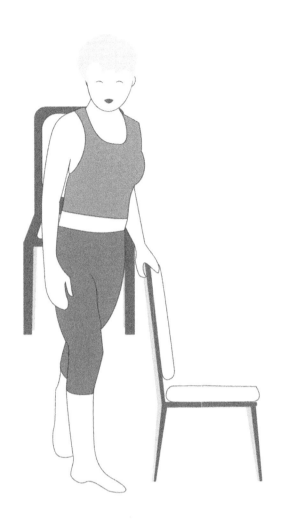

Another thing that's really important that you work on is adding unpredictable elements to it. So not knowing what's coming is another way to challenge your balance.

It's hard to do that by yourself, but in sessions, what I would do is I would wait until the last minute, and if my client was doing this and I'd either say right or left or forward, and that means they either need to step to the right or they need to step forward, or they need to step to the left. And again, takes more of the thinking out of it, which is really important when these situations come up in real life.

That is why, if you have the opportunity, you can perform this exercise with the help of someone who gives you the movement instructions at the last moment. You will see, as well as use it will be a lot of fun doing it together!

So there are a lot of different directions. This can go the main point of this exercise. Again, I wanna just reiterate it's that immediate step that you take after you stand up from a chair; you want that to be as automatic as possible, where you have to do the least amount of thinking.

Remember, there are a lot of situations that come up where you're either rushed, or you're thinking about something else. So these scenarios or that step needs to be automatic. So the best way to get that more automatic is to practice, practice, practice when you're not distracted, or you're not actually in a rush to make sure that you are safe, and then hopefully, eventually, the end goal be being that that's gonna become more automatic.

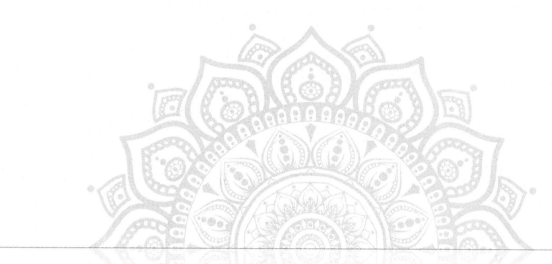

SO I HOPE YOU ENJOYED THESE SIMPLE EXERCISES AS MUCH AS I DID!

NOW THAT YOU KNOW YOUR BODY BETTER, LET'S DISCOVER TOGETHER EVERYTHING YOU CAN DO TO TRAIN YOUR BALANCE BY BUILDING STRENGTH AND CONFIDENCE INSIDE AND OUTSIDE YOU!

*If you're enjoying this book,
I'd love to read your honest Amazon review!*

Chapter 7
Getting Ready

Warming up

To be carried out correctly, every balance session for seniors must be preceded by an adequate period of warming up the body.

5-10 minutes of slow walking is often enough to prepare the body and muscles for physical activity. Warming up, in fact, allows you to activate the muscles in order to prepare them for subsequent physical activity, reducing the risk of muscle tears.

Here are two movements helpful for this purpose.

1. <u>March your feet in place</u>

Keeping your back straight and sitting or standing (depending on your strength and balance skills), march your feet, lifting them alternately, for three to five minutes to increase core body temperature and prepare the muscles and joints.

If you are successful and do not lose your balance, draw large circles with your arms as you march.

2. <u>Ankle circles</u>

Make circles with the ankles to activate the core and loosen the ankle joints. At this point, you can start with the actual training to challenge your balance.

Balance exercises equipments for home workouts

Several tools allow the person to work on this skill for those who are starting to train balance. There are both specific tools dedicated exclusively to improving the ability to stay balanced and multifunctional tools to be used for this purpose.

In this case, I am entering them for informational purposes only so that you know that there is a level of 'help' to expand your practice's knowledge. However, for this book, we will only use the most important tool: your body!

Let's discover the main tools to perform balance exercises.

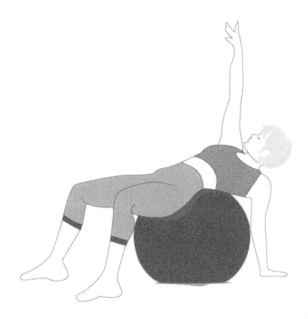

• Fitness Ball: to carry out balance exercises, the fitness ball is a very versatile and interesting tool. It is a non-slip PVC ball, easy to inflate and carry, with which to perform various exercises, including pilates, yoga, and posture improvement.

• Bosu: have you ever heard of exercises with the Bosu? It is a rubber hemisphere designed to improve balance, strength, and endurance. A fitness accessory that works all body muscles: it tones the abdomen, arms, and legs, improving aesthetics and

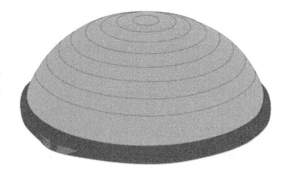

accelerating recovery from sprains and trauma. The tool is suitable for people in good physical condition, without injuries or disabilities. The best way to take advantage of this fitness accessory is to get advice from an instructor; an expert person will be able to identify the exercises that best suit your needs, as well as guide the execution of the activities so that no accidents occur.

Dizziness-related issues

More than a third of the population over 65 is affected by balance disorders, acutely or chronically. We said it and stole it. The figure is constantly increasing and involves frequent use of various health facilities. And it all comes from dizziness.
Vertigo, in the elderly, is responsible for both immediate effects, such as traumatic falls, and long-term effects, such as chronic postural dysfunctions, subjective insecurity, and fear to the point of anguish with the consequent impairment of usual life activities.

The elderly patient often presents agitated due to associated, severe, and disturbing autonomic symptoms such as nausea, vomiting, sweating, and tachycardia. Sometimes they report these signs with great confusion, supported and amplified by anxiety.

The possible co-presence of a clinical picture of depression, previous or secondary to the disorder, makes it difficult to reduce the alarm thus created.

And there is also a low sensitivity to this type of discomfort due to an inadequate general ability to manage a complex psycho-bodily problem that alters the person's quality of life in terms of loss of calm, reduction of active mobility, and general of its global autonomy.

Here are some simple and effective remedies to reduce vertigo that lead to falling.

- In the case of poor circulation, a natural remedy is the use of the Ginko Biloba plant because of its properties of stimulating blood circulation and, in particular, producing the vessels in the brain with better oxygen supply to the brain. This leads to considerably reduced dizziness if the triggering cause is a reduction in blood flow at the capillary level.

- Another home remedy is the use of ginger in the form of an infusion to be drunk several times a day. We can grate this spicy root in hot water and sip the herbal tea after a few moments. This plant also has properties of blood circulation stimulation resulting in a decrease in the sense of dizziness.

- An essential element to be included and balanced in one's diet to promote the removal of dizziness is the contribution of magnesium. This mineral supports the oxygenation of the muscles and is, therefore, very important for movement and walking. Foods that contain reasonable amounts of magnesium are figs, spinach, artichokes, walnuts, pumpkin sprouts, dates, and brown rice.
- I once used a home remedy made with vinegar to dull the sense of vertigo, mainly when it was associated with nausea. It was enough to soak a handkerchief or cotton in the vinegar and rub it on the temples. In this way, the smell of vinegar soothed the discomforts of that moment of both nausea and dizziness.

- We can treat dizziness generated by stress, anxiety, and panic attacks using plants with calming and relaxing properties. Among these plants, we remember lemon balm, passion flower, lavender, and chamomile. The form to take them can be the infusion to be sipped several times a day, taking some time to relax.

- Furthermore, lemon balm and lavender can be used as essential oils to be dispersed in the environment and inhaled when needed.

- Finally, the treatments of kinesiology, foot reflexology, relaxation techniques, and manipulation treatments are indicated to relax and disperse tension, especially at the muscular level.

- If the attacks of dizziness are powerful, it is good to go to bed in a quiet environment and with little light to stop dizziness and lower nausea related to vertigo.

- When dizziness is frequent and intense, it is good to consult a doctor to verify that the problem originates inside the ear. In this case, the doctor will usually intervene with particular medicines.

Postures to reduce dizziness

I am obliged to repeat this: the vertiginous syndrome associated with labyrinthitis must be preceded by a careful diagnosis that concerns all the receptors in our body and which are involved in cases of labyrinthitis; ear, sight, and neurological examinations will then be carried out.
However, some exercises can help relieve symptoms effectively. Here are a few.

Stability ball and proprioception
First, the body's internal balance must be rearranged, which often requires continuous proprioceptive training over time. Not small exercises, not random and disordered sequences but an actual work program with stability balls, tools, and work on the ground with a mat.

Re-education of Semont and Brandt Daroff with physiotherapy
There is real physiotherapy, and it is done first in the presence of a doctor or physiotherapist.
After sitting sideways on the bed, one quickly gets onto the left side and waits for vertigo to end. If you don't feel dizzy, stay in the position for 30 seconds. Then you return to the sitting place and hold it for 30 seconds or until the dizziness is exhausted. You pass with a certain speed on the right side, and if there is no vertigo, you maintain the position.
You should repeat these exercises every 3 hours and stop if dizziness does not appear beyond two days.

Visualization + breathing

To mitigate these sensations of anxiety and dizziness, it is necessary to work with a certain constancy in the direction of 'seeing with our inner eyes.' The exercise is an actual practice, not too complex, but it requires concentration and a suitable space for execution.
Sit the straight column and the pelvis aligned with the chest, and bring your hands up.
You can turn your face left and right by observing the movement of your breathing.
These poses calm the mind and are effective if you avoid performing them too quickly.
Breathing exercise alone helps. You can also associate a visualization of a wave coming in and retracting or an expansion of colors under the chest and inside the belly spread out to the head. Alternatively, a beam of light radiates from the cervical to the head and goes downwards. Finally, at home, you can practice classic pranayama exercises in combination with the asanas that allow the whole system to take root on the ground.

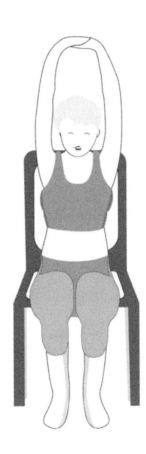

Chapter 8
Targeted exercises to boost your strength, posture, and flexibility

STANDING EXERCISES FOR FALLING PREVENTION

To train in this sense, you can use a series of balance exercises at home, without special equipment, but simply a free body.

The methodology of these exercises is to be performed in unstable conditions to activate the attention of your body and those receptors we have discussed.

This type of training should be at least 1-2 times a week, making sure that it becomes a routine and stable appointment to effectively intervene on your balance.

STAND ON ONE LEG

Bend the leg forward or backward and remain standing on the other leg for as long as possible.

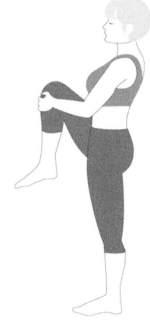

How it becomes more difficult:
• Move the bent leg alternately forwards and backward;
• Close eyes;
• Tilt your head back;
• Keeping your eyes closed, tilt your head back while.

STANDING POSITION WITH FEET ALIGNED

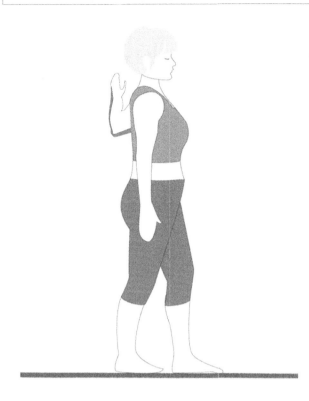

Place the foot in front of the foot on which the weight rests so that the front foot's heel touches the toes of the rear foot. Hold the position as long as possible.

How it becomes more difficult:
•Close eyes;
•Tilt your head back;
• While closing your eyes, tilt your head back;
•Place your foot behind the foot on which the weight rests.

STAND ON YOUR TOES

Stand with both feet on your toes and try to maintain the position for as long as possible.

So it becomes more difficult:
• Spring up by lowering and raising your heels;
• Tiptoe on one leg;
• Stand with one leg on tiptoe on a rolled-up pillow or blanket.

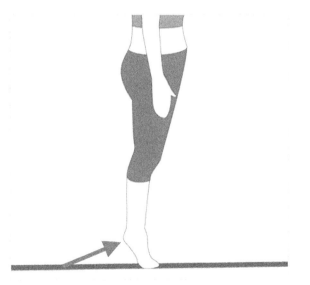

218

RAISE THE LEG TO THE SIDE

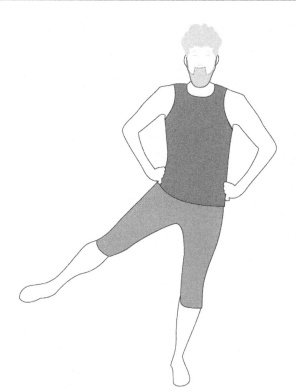

Stand and put the weight of your body on one leg. Then lift the other leg laterally as much as possible, keeping the torso always in an upright position.

How it becomes more difficult:
•Move the raised leg forward, sideways, and backward without touching the ground;
•Do the same exercise keeping your eyes closed.

LUNGE

Step forward with one leg, and step back with the other leg. Lower the pelvis until the knee of the front leg forms a right angle. Straighten up and repeat the exercise.

How it becomes more difficult:
• Place your front foot, back foot, or both feet on a pillow or rolled blanket;
• Decrease the distance between the feet;
• Close eyes.

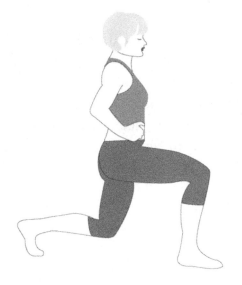

SINGLE OR DOUBLE LEG SQUAT

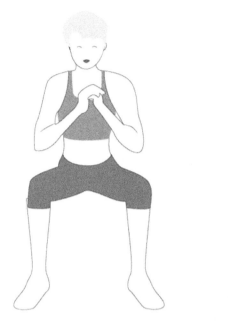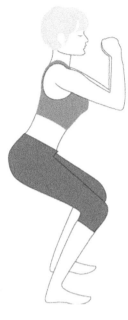

A very simple and well-known exercise is the Single Leg Squat, the version of one leg of the famous squat exercise.

Put your hands on your hips and keep your torso straight, then keep one leg slightly raised and lower your torso by bending the other leg.

Repeat the exercise for an equal number of repetitions for both legs.

Alternatively, you can perform the normal squat.

LUNGE TO FRONT KICK

Standing upright and staring forward, step back with one leg, straighten it and bend the knee to the ground, then stand up and straighten the leg forward as if to give a kick. The arms must follow the movement of the body.

Then repeat the exercise on the other leg as well.

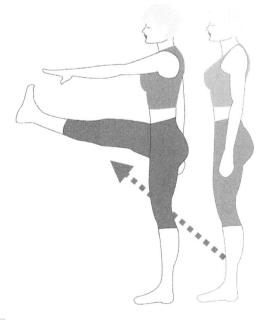

EYE MOVEMENT

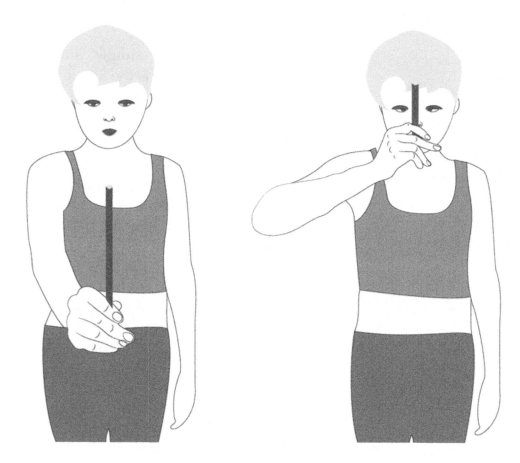

On a wall, stick a sheet of paper with written text and put about 25 centimeters apart. Slowly from left to right, move your head trying to keep the letters on the paper in focus. Perform this exercise for a minute, pause and repeat by moving your head from top to bottom.

To facilitate the execution, without losing effectiveness, you can repeat the exercise using an object. Take it in your hand and bring it to a distance equal to your arm. Then look at the object and move it from right to left or back and forth, following it with your gaze.

By performing these exercises, it will be normal to see a difference in yield and ease of movement between the limbs involved. Very often, it is more difficult to stay on one leg rather than the other, and all this is not a problem or cause for alarm, but only that it is advisable to continue training to improve your overall balance.

SEATED EXERCISES FOR FALLING PREVENTION

SEATED TRUNK MOVEMENT 1

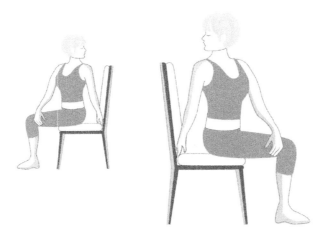

Sit on the edge of the chair.
Gently rotate the shoulders from one side to the other.

Repeat 20 times.

SEATED TRUNK MOVEMENT 2

I only recommend this exercise for those with no
back pain.
Position: Seated on the chair.

Lean forward to grab an object that is on the
ground.

Fold over to put the object back on the ground.
Repeat 20 times.

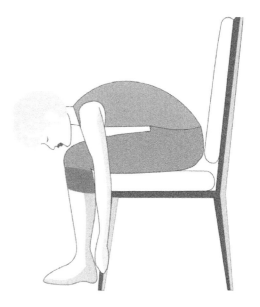

FOSTER'S MANEUVER

The Foster maneuver is one of the easiest to perform because it does not require lying down or the help of another person.

It will be necessary to proceed as follows:
- Kneel on a comfortable surface and place your hands on the floor, moving your head up and down (especially if you feel dizzy);
- Then, bring your head to the ground, trying to touch your knees;
- Without lifting the head from the ground, rotate it 45 degrees towards the side of the affected ear, looking towards the shoulder. Maintain this position for 30 seconds;
- With your head rotated 45 degrees, bring it to shoulder height;
- Stay in this position for 30 seconds;
- Raise your head to the normal position.

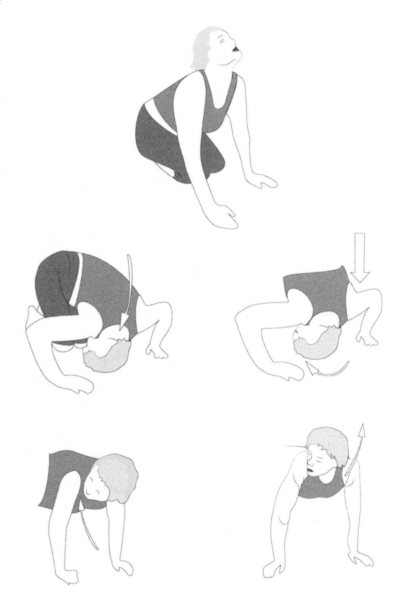

It is necessary to repeat the maneuver three to five times with a 15-minute break between one repetition and the next.

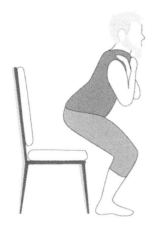 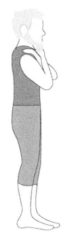

Sit in the front chair, feet firmly anchored to the ground.
Define the angle of the pelvis according to the desired load: pelvis upright position = less resistance / pelvis position bent forward = stronger resistance.

Put your arms crossed in front of the chest or placed on the hips.

Slowly bend the lumbar and thoracic spine forward (rotate it inwards) and straighten it again. The pelvis remains fixed during the exercise. Breathe out while straightening.

Depending on the angle of the pelvis chosen, keep the torso more or less bent forward; the pelvis, hips, and knees are in the same starting position.

STRAIGHTENING OF THE TRUNK - STANDING VARIANT (MORE DIFFICULT)

Perform the same exercise standing up. Standing, pelvis-width legs, feet parallel, buttock muscles consciously taut, pelvis stable.

Attention: Stabilizing the pelvis and the angle of the hips and knees during exercise is an arduous task. It is, therefore, necessary to explain the individual phases of the practice continuously and for different training units, instructing the participants precisely and controlling the position!

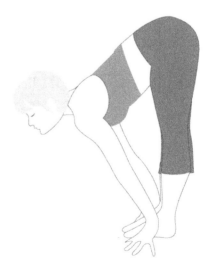

WALKING EXERCISES FOR FALLING PREVENTION

Balance is a prerequisite for many daily motor activity tasks, including the biological activity of walking. Even if we are unaware, walking requires specific postural stability and the innate ability to maintain balance. And only a child knows how challenging it can be!

Let's remember some basic rules of walking naturally:

- Engaging in moving the center of gravity of the body (forward, backward, sideways, downward, upward);
- Perceiving the points of support (heel-sole-toes);
- Varying the position of the feet while walking (on the heels, on the tips of the toes, on the outer side of the feet);
- Changing of direction, making turns;
- Changing your pace (e.g., starting or stopping abruptly at robotic speed, lifting your knee higher, etc.);
- Accentuating the right or left step (alternating, in rhythm);
- Walking on a rope, a stick, a hoof, an edge, a line, etc.;
- Walking to the rhythm of music or different rhythms (e.g. 'off-beat rhythm'), or synchronizing the combination of tasks with the sequence of steps;
- with your eyes, directing your gaze to visual targets (e.g., a person in the immediate vicinity, the following object with a particular color, etc.);
- with the upper extremities, performing other movements on various levels (e.g., writing names in the air, clapping hands, drawing eights in the air, etc.);
- hold (in balance), throwing or dribbling everyday objects (tray with glass), or other entities (ball, ball, handkerchief, etc.);
- Duoing with a partner (e.g., following your partner, throwing a ball, etc.);
- Holding a stick at both ends and performing perturbing stimuli on the same (from a partner);
- combination of a motor and cognitive component (e.g., placing obstacles in the path).

In short, if this natural security and the basis for doing so are removed, even the simple act of walking becomes a nightmare!

Fortunately, there are some fun exercises to do it carefully and consciously!

WALK CLOSE TO A WALL, HEEL TO TOE

Stand arm's length from the wall (close enough that you can touch it for light support if needed) and turn around so that one shoulder is adjacent to the wall.

Step forward with the left foot, so the left heel is just in front of the toe of the right foot.

Continue walking like this (like on a balance beam) until you have managed to walk the length of the wall.

If this exercise is too easy, increase the difficulty by walking backward. Cross your arms over your chest, then close your eyes or turn your head from side to side while walking.

To make things even more complicated, introduce a cognitive challenge, such as counting backward from 100 in increments of 3 while walking. Fun, isn't it? :)

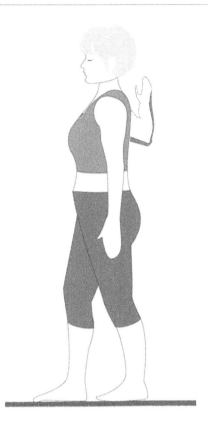

WALK ON A ROPE

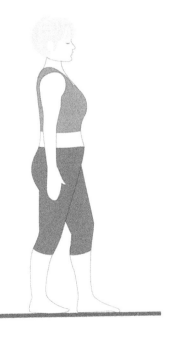

Calm down, I'm not telling you to tie a piece of string to two poles and be a tightrope walker! We are still at floor level!

Alternatively, you can lay a string or tape on the floor or put adhesive on the floor. The important thing, in fact, is to draw a straight line.

Keeping your hands on your hips, walk back and forth following the line, never 'falling' to the side.

Continue for 1 minute.

'NOVICE' WALKING

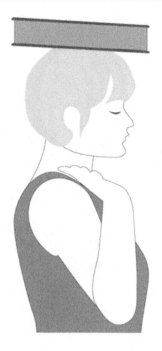

Stand upright with a pillow, a book, or a newspaper resting on your head.

Walk in a straight line, trying to maintain posture and balance so that the object does not fall.

Then try to circle or walk in a zigzag, moving backward or from side to side, depending on your health situation.

Continue for about 1 minute.

LET'S CARDIO

Continuous and modulated exercise generates positive physiological changes in our body; we know that. But, of course, remember to respect your health and body by doing these cardio exercises if you feel like it. Do not stress the body, and do not stress yourself!

- Dance is not about performing a choreography but a routine that works the back muscles. Raise one leg, lower it and lift the other: 20 reps and switch legs;
- Free Jumps: perform 15 seconds of jumps. Rest for 30 seconds. Then repeat the sequence 3 times;
- Up and down on the stairs: do a series of 20 repetitions, and increase the intensity to accelerate the pulse. After 6 minutes, if you start with the right leg, start again from the left

And if you particularly liked the stairs (right? :)), in the next chapter you will discover a whole flow to train your balance and prevent falls thanks to the stairs!

Chapter 9
Stair Flow

Always remember to perform this flow with your sneakers or running shoes. Don't do it wearing socks, because it can be very slippery!

1. UP AND DOWN RIGHT FOOT

The first exercise goes up on the right foot and down on the right foot. You must have a handrailing to do this exercise, so you don't lose your balance. So let's do it.

You're going to notice that if you do this, you are using more muscles in the front of the tight.

You can do this couple of times up and down, all on the right side, until you get fatigued.

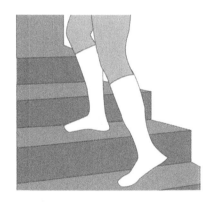

Repeat two times up to five: you will 1otice that the more you practice, the more it'll take longer for you to get fatigued.

2. UP AND DOWN LEFT FOOT

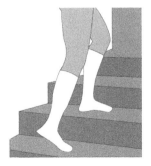

So exercise number two is the same, but now with the left leg.

So you will go up and down, always starting with the left leg.

Try to keep your body straight, holding on to the handrail.

You can do this up and down a couple of times: if you have stairs at home, that's a great exercise to start your day

3. SIDEWAYS UP AND DOWN RIGHT FOOT

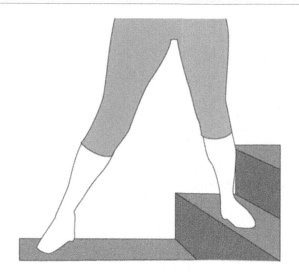

Exercise three is on the side. We are not going to go all the way up. We are just going to go one step. If you feel that you're going to lose your balance, you can hold on to the handrail, but usually, this is not a problem.

So on your right side, you're going to go one step down. If you are new to this, you may feel tired on the side of your thighs.

Repeat ten times and then increase to 20.

4. SIDEWAYS UP AND DOWN LEFT FOOT

Number four is on the other side.

Go sideways up and down with the left foot.

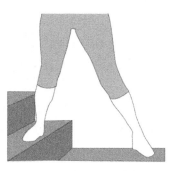

Sometimes you need to look at where you are, but once you get used to this exercise, you can look straight, and you don't even need to look at the step again.

5. BACKWARDS TOUCH RIGHT FOOT

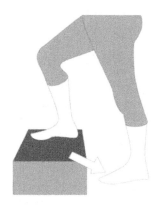

The following exercise is backward. We need to exercise the glute muscles, which are used so weak, and strengthen them. This is an excellent strengthening exercise.

You're going to step on the first step here, and you're going to touch and come back. So we are going to do this first with the right foot. Repeat it eight times. With time, you can increase it to 12 -20.

6. BACKWARDS TOUCH LEFT FOOT

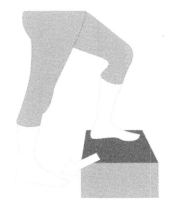

Now repeat the previous exercise with the left foot.

Step on the first step and just touch the ground; then touch and come back. Repeat it eight times.

With time, you can increase it to 12 -20.

7. SIDEWAYS RIGHT SIDE

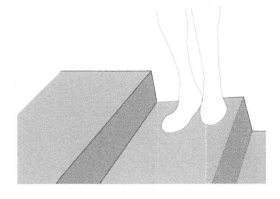

The upcoming exercise also involves touching. Stay on the floor with one foot, but now on the side. Now you're going to stay only on the first step and touch and come back to life before.

It's a good strengthening and balance exercise: touching the tip of your tip toes on the side forces your other leg to be strong and to hold your balance. Repeat it eight times.

8. SIDEWAYS LEFT SIDE

Perform the previous exercise on the left side, starting with eight repetitions.

You can increase them to 12 and 20.

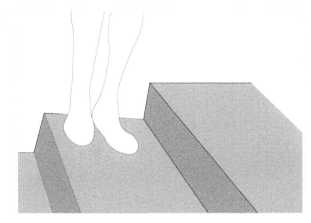

9. HEELS STRETCHING

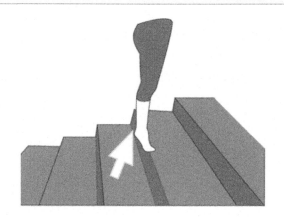 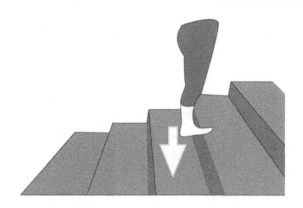

So the following two exercises are our final stretching. We will stretch the plantar fascia and the muscles on the back of our leg.

We're going to step on the edge of the first stair step and just go down, both feet together but without the heels touching the floor. You can feel that all of the back of the leg is stretching.

Sometimes we have muscle cramps on the back of our legs, which is an excellent exercise to prevent muscle cramps. When doing this final stretch, it is always advisable to lean against the handrail.

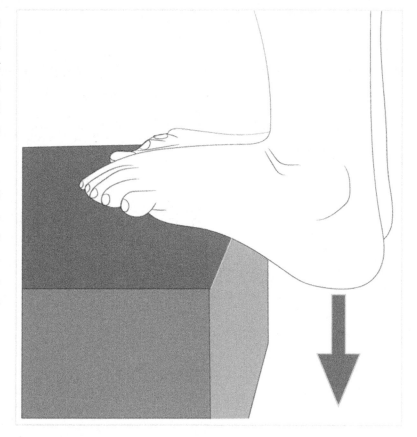

10. HAMSTRINGS STRETCHING BOTH SIDES

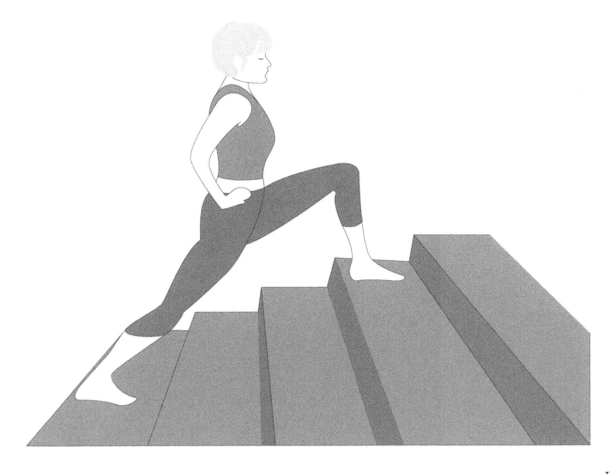

In the last exercise of this routine, we will stretch all the muscles of the back of the thigh, the knee, and the back of the leg.

If you're not used to doing this, you can use the second step and try to touch the tip of your foot with your hand. Or maybe you can then go on to the third step. So touch your tiptoes and stretch, stretch, stretch, on both sides!

Try to also stretch all your back muscles, lowering your head.

And remember: do not force your hand, do not seek perfection, but rather focus on the general feeling of well-being, strength, and stability that you will find day after day!

BOOK 5:
WATER AEROBICS AND LOW-IMPACT SWIMMING POOL EXERCISES FOR SENIORS

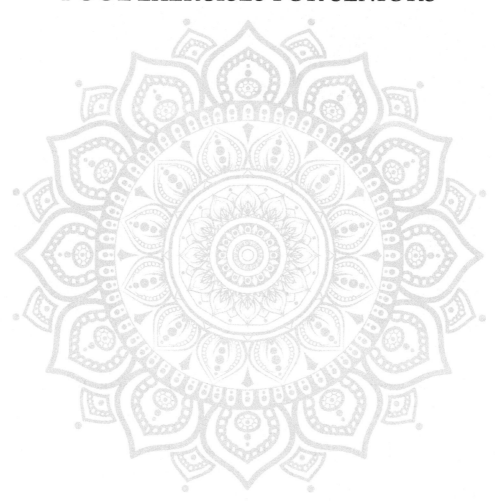

Chapter 1
Light and Alive

On summer days, nothing is more pleasant than a dip in the sea or the pool. Swimming tones the body, while floating relaxes the mind and clears it of negative thoughts.

This is also why swimming and exercising in the water are one of the oldest physical activities.

The first evidence dated back to 7,000 years ago and was found in Egypt, in the so-called Swimmers' Cave, on whose walls human figures practice swimming are engraved. From historical sources, we know that swimming was then of great importance to the Greeks and Romans. The philosopher Plato argued that it should be an essential part of education.

Even today, it is considered one of the complete sports activities to stay healthy, without any age limit. It is recommended for children to promote their harmonious development, for adults to maintain the efficiency of the motor system and for seniors to reduce the incidence of cardiovascular diseases and combat osteoarthritis. But that is not all. In recent times, in fact, research has identified a natural link between swimming and longevity.

According to a study conducted by South California University (USA), those who choose to practice swimming have a risk of death even lower than 50% compared to those who prefer walking or running or those who do not practice any sport. The research lasted 32 years and was conducted on 40,000 individuals between the ages of 20 and 90, all practicing different sports.

Exercising in water is a helpful discipline to improve both physical fitness and the body's well-being. Furthermore, being a low-impact sport, it has the advantage of not straining the lower joints as intensely as running and walking and is suitable for those suffering from mobility problems or other chronic disorders - such as arthritis - which can affect the ability to carry out the exercise. Water reduces the pressure on the body, supporting its weight and absorbing shocks.

This does not mean that you should stop running or walking! On the other hand, I'm the first who loves running in the morning, when the sky shines with the first rays of the rising sun … However, studies such as the Californian one provide extra motivation for those who are already water lovers or those who think that it is never too late to learn something new.

Learning, trying, feeling light and alive ... isn't this the elixir of life? I think so. Especially from such a joyful activity that brings with it many benefits for our health at every age, with a 'senior' eye that should not be underestimated!

Chapter 2
Benefits of Low-Impact Water Aerobics

The therapeutic effects of water and swimming on elderly people are, therefore, multiple, as confirmed by many studies.

One of the most reliable is from the Harvard Medicine School, according to which performing water aerobics for at least 30-45 minutes promotes an increase in heart rate and improves heart health, reducing the risk of heart attack and stroke. In addition, after a few minutes of entering the water, blood pressure is reduced, while the surrounding temperature and the position, prone or supine, promote blood circulation through peripheral vasodilation. Finally, thanks to the buoyancy thrust, the water also makes large movements of the extremities possible, particularly beneficial for counteracting the effects of arthrosis.

But there is another good reason to practice water and low-impact exercises in gold age, which is related to the decrease in muscle function, a phenomenon known as sarcopenia. The problem is not insignificant; it concerns 5-13% of people between 60 and 70 years, reaching 11-50% of the over-80s.

Swimming, however, is not only a commitment and effort but also a way to stay healthy while having fun. Soft water programs for seniors that include group lessons offer new opportunities for meeting and socializing, with predictable positive effects on mood.

Practicing aerobic exercises, moreover, helps improve sleep - and therefore the quality of life - even when you are no longer young. Being a demanding exercise for the muscles, it produces a physiological sense of fatigue in those who practice it, favored by the natural relaxation induced by contact with water.

So let's find out in detail all the main benefits of water aerobics for the elderly.

<u>Lightness and simplicity</u>
Performing the exercises in the water seems more straightforward because the water makes the body light, but the resistance it generates leads the muscles to perform very intense work. That's why it is one of the most widespread fitness activities, both for the high fun rate and for the satisfaction of seeing the first results after the first sessions. The

constant water massage immediately makes the skin more toned and smooth. But the benefits for your general mood do not end up here.

Beating the heat
The first obvious benefit of water aerobics is to make it possible to train even in scorching temperatures. In addition to a series of beneficial effects, water allows you to always stay calm and not suffer from the symptoms of fatigue and heat.

Water resistance makes training more effective and enjoyable
The movements of a body immersed in water encounter a resistance 12 times higher than that of air. The toning effect is more significant and faster. While having fun, you burn more calories than the same dry workout. But doing physical activity in the water also leads to an improvement in the mood because it facilitates the production of endorphins. You are more serene and satisfied.

Intense work made easy
The physical effort required by movements and exercises performed at low intensity over a prolonged period meets the resistance force of water. If, on the one hand, the water does not reveal the physical effort that underlies the movements, on the other, it requires more intense work from a muscular point of view.

Water gymnastics gets your body in motion
Aquatic training helps fight water retention and cellulite because it favors the exchange of liquids. Your body will be more harmonious and responsive in a few sessions. You will not have to feel the annoying sensation caused by lactic acid, which is usually a sentence when you perform traditional physical activities.

Preserve joint health
When you feel overweight and start exercising, your legs can be affected, as they have to support a heavier body in stressful activities. Therefore, water training is especially recommended for those with a few extra pounds: you can train without risk, and the impact on the knee joints is minimal. In addition, it improves posture and promotes the ability to balance.

Stretching of the muscles
Aquaerobics, like any other water sport, promotes the progressive stretching of the muscles. The same aerobic exercises practiced out of the water favor muscle enlargement and definition. That's why doing it is so good!

Full Body training

The water aerobics training session lasts between 30 and 45 minutes and asks the body to get used to working at 50% or 60% of maximum heart rate with a background run, arm exercises, leg movements, and exercises for the buttocks.

To summon up, low-impact water aerobics exercises:

• Improve muscular strength;

• Increase flexibility;

• Enhance cardiovascular fitness;

• Alleviate pain;

• Rehabilitate injuries;

• Make you stay healthy.

Intensity modulation

Water aerobics is less intense from a physical point of view than the variant performed on land. You can also adjust it to different levels of difficulty based on the intensity of the movements indicated and the height of the water.

It goes without saying that one can do the exercises with water that reaches waist or chest height or with high water that requires training in buoyancy mode.

Draining effect

The pressure of the water works on the tissues, and the various exercises produce currents that develop a massaging action on the body. Many activities include training in the pool to enhance the anti-cellulite effect: there are hydro bike exercises to fight cellulite, aquafitness or aqua aerobics against orange peel.

The constant water massage generates a draining and remodeling action on the tissues able to relax, improve the aesthetic appearance and manage the problems of the circulatory system (e.g., cellulite, stagnation of liquids, swollen legs, and so on).

It's good for the heart

Another great aspect of water gymnastics is that the resistance provided by the water, combined with rapid movements, keeps the heart in training without excessive effort. So, when you are exercising it, and like any other muscle, the more you train your heart, the stronger it gets.

Therefore, water exercises, such as water aerobics, help the cardiovascular system and reduce hypertension.

It acts on the metabolism

When a body is immersed in water, body temperature drops. The body is therefore forced to produce more calories taken from adipose tissue.

Additionally, the acceleration of metabolism corresponds to the increase in aerobic activity, consequent improvement in physical fitness.

Relaxation

The movements in the water are marked by the rhythm of the background music and accompanied by group dances, a mix that allows the training to be perceived as a water game and gives an unparalleled sense of mental relief.

Doctors recommend it

In conclusion, swimming can be considered a sport suitable (almost) for everyone. Before starting, however, it is always useful to undergo a medical check-up, especially for cardiovascular or respiratory diseases. Just as it is essential to avoid 'do it yourself,' evaluating the most appropriate training methods without running risks. For example, in case of back pain, hip problems, or a herniated disc, it is preferable to avoid the frog style. In a group or alone, water exercises are good for you for rehabilitation or fitness.

It is crucial to do it under the guidance of qualified and safe instructors, especially in the beginning of the practise.

Specific benefits for seniors

The combination of exercise and water action develops significant benefits for seniors in water aerobics and other low-impact disciplines developed with the body immersed in water.

Why is it so good to do water aerobics if you are living your senior years?

- Limiting trauma: the body in the water weighs 10% less than the weight on the ground, and this reduces stress on the muscles and joints;
- Facilitating movement: the sense of lightness imparted by the water makes it easier to perform the required exercises;
- Toning the muscles: the presence of water prompts the body to use all the muscles to maintain balance and carry out the sequence;
- Burning calories: the aerobic process is also carried out in water due to the type of training and the resistance strength of the water. The body first consumes glycogen stores and then switches to fat stores to support the pace;

- Improving circulation: the water currents create a massage that affects venous circulation and counteracts various problems.
- Infusing relaxation: water promotes muscle relaxation, relieves pain, and creates a fun environment that relieves tension.

Training in the water is, ultimately, the perfect union of every single activity that we have discovered together in the course of this book. Each muscle 'conspires' so that you boost your strength, your stability, and your balance for an active and happy life!

And now... let's take (water) action!

Chapter 3
Types of Water Exercises

What are the most practiced exercises in the water? The most popular is undoubtedly water aerobics, followed by swimming and the water treadmill and hydro bikes. Different tools and accessories are used in each of these activities.

Water Aerobics

Water aerobics is the most popular gymnastics, especially among women. It is the simple transposition in the water of disciplines that are generally practiced in the gym (e.g., Aerobics and step). The accessories used for this sport are many:

- weights;
- belts;
- tubes;
- step;
- bikes;
- tapis roulant.

In some activities (such as bikes and tapis roulant), the body must be totally immersed in water to prevent it from cooling down. Clothing must also comply with the training location, that is, the water. Green light to practical costumes, headphones, and earplugs (if you suffer from otitis).

In more experienced athletes, supports are often applied to the wrists and ankles that are able to move larger quantities of water, allowing the subject to intensify sports activity and strengthen the biceps, quadriceps, shoulders, and adductors.

Aquawalking

An alternative to water aerobics is aqua walking, or walking in the water that replaces that on the road but maintains (if it does not increase them) the typical benefits of the walk. The practice of aqua walking is practiced above all by young people who make it a natural fashion.

The walk in the water can be performed with the aid of a snare mat to make the legs more toned and firm the buttocks. The activity is made more enjoyable and engaging thanks to the help of comfortable headphones for listening to good music.

Aquastep

This practice is the variant of water aerobics with the difference that instead of being carried out free body, it is supported by a step or platform (as is done in classic gyms). This platform is fixed to the bottom of the pool by means of suction cups. Exercise requires a lot of physical effort and allows you to stimulate the abdominals, thighs, and buttocks.

While in the step on the ground, the movement must oppose the force of gravity (whose direction goes from top to bottom), in the water, all actions must counteract the buoyancy force (bottom to top) and therefore oppose the 'currents' they themselves created. It is thanks to the resistance opposed by the water that there is a greater calorie expenditure and more significant muscular effort. In this way, weight loss and complete muscle toning are promoted.

For advanced

Hydrospinning

If you want to try the experience of cycling and to pedal in the water, the hydro bike course is for you.

Hydrobike or hydrospinning is a sport that is practiced exclusively in water with simple and articulated exercise bikes. It is called hydrospinning precisely because it recalls spinning exercises combined with those of the traditional exercise bike to the rhythm of the music. The bike used is made of steel with comfortable and non-slip saddles.

The hydro bike combines various types of exercises for the arms as well. It is, in fact, possible to make movements with the arms, even using floating dumbbells which help to concentrate the effort on the muscles of the arms leaving the backlight.

The practice is suitable for those who want to lose weight or are not too inclined to sports. It is a sport that trains the body but does it with fun.

Aquafitness

This discipline represents the evolution of water aerobics. The exercises that are performed are similar; the difference is in the resistance offered by the new workout. Acquafitness is practiced with supports that can be applied to the ankles and wrists that have side flaps and are used to increase the intensity of work. Applied to the legs, they are helpful for increasing the strength of the quadriceps (with forwarding leg movements).

Many choose to follow the acquafitness courses, considered more complete and more intense from the point of view of training. Numerous courses are spreading to become an instructor of water aerobics and all disciplines related to this sport.

Aquatraining

This particular activity is very popular with lovers of physical activity and 'suspension' sports.

Aquatraining consists of a particular training performed in buoyancy with unique belts so as not to touch the bottom of the pool (but to stay afloat).

The pace of work varies continuously and is only interspersed with a few exercises out of the water (performed by the pool for a few minutes) and then back in the water. Aquatraining is a practice suitable for those who already have strengthened core muscles and excellent physical endurance.

Chapter 4
Safety Tips Before Starting

General Rules

As we have mentioned many times, the water aerobics exercises to perform are, in most cases, straightforward and low impact. And for this reason, they can be practiced by practically everyone, even if they have not been physically active for some time.

The exciting thing is that, being in the water, anyone who practices can independently decide the intensity of the effort to be applied, customizing the training according to their physical conditions without overloading.

Before starting, therefore, here is what you need to know and how you can prepare yourself for this new wellness challenge and love for yourself!

- To get the best results from water gymnastics, it is essential to be constant, but this obviously also applies to all types of physical exercise to be carried out in or out of the water. With a frequency of two training sessions a week, the first results will not be long in coming, while those who can train three times will immediately notice the first benefits already from the second week.

- Water aerobics does not just mean constancy and dedication because the effort will also be rewarded in terms of mood. As with other forms of physical activity, movement helps the body to produce endorphins, hormones responsible for good mood. Unlike other sports, however, doing aqua aerobics is fun for the type of exercises performed, which can also be performed with the help of friendly tools to be used in the water.

- Water Aerobics is also strongly recommended for those suffering from back and muscle pains generated by being overweight, incorrect postures, and more or less severe contractures.

Staying Safe in the Water

Among the tips to consider when you want to start water aerobics, there are certain to consider well the time you have available, why you want to swim regularly, when you can swim during the day, and other essential points.

Why starting in the first place?
Motivation is essential, and it must be evident right away. It is not enough to say, 'I'm going to swim in the pool to keep fit a little,' because then you risk going around in circles without appreciable consequences and, over time, with less and less motivation. So before packing your bag and entering a swimming pool, it is good to have clear your goal.

To get distracted and have fun? Release stress? Lose weight? Improve the technique? Improve performance? Tone your muscles?

Each one of these goals asks for a different approach, from the freedom to go when you can and have time to enroll in a course or be followed by a coach.

Clear goals = great motivation.

How many times can I go?
The time available greatly influences the achievement of our goals. Being able to go to the pool only once a week, you can't think of improving your style or times but of having fun and letting off some steam.

Likewise, going to the pool three times a week just to soak would be a waste of time, and then it would be worth trying to do something more.

Similarly, with less than 3 hours a week available for swimming, it is difficult to think about losing weight by swimming or toning up your muscles. Then you must be content with releasing a little stress and tension without paying too much attention to the mirror and scales.

From what level do I start?
Your starting level also has a lot of influence on expectations and, consequently, on gratification and satisfaction. If you start from scratch, that is, not only have you never swam regularly but not even anything else to keep fit, know that yes, swimming has many advantages, but you will still need perseverance and tenacity to be able to train regularly and for distances sufficient for your remise en forme.

Or you go back to swimming after a long pause or injury, and then the head tells you something, but the body reacts in another way, and you have to arm yourself with a lot of patience to find your automatisms.

Do I have the right equipment?

Of all the things you can pack to go to the pool, in the end, three things are significant in terms of equipment: goggles, cap, and swimsuit. Not that it is necessary to spend immediately for the top of the range, but knowing how real goggles are made for swimming in the pool, how to choose a comfortable cap, and which swimsuit to use is already a good starting point to avoid losing patience.

What about the water temperature?

The ideal temperature of a swimming pool can vary depending on its use. For example, if children or seniors use the pool, a heated one is recommended. In any case, the ideal temperature is between 78 and 82 Fahrenheit (26-28° Celsius).

Know how to swim

Even if the purpose of water aerobics is not to become swimming champions, it is always helpful to know the principles of this noble discipline in order to get the most out of training.

Breathing, moving, and managing the unexpected in the water, in fact, is an extra weapon to relax, knowing you know the 'rules of the game.' Before starting with the low-impact routine in the water, therefore, talk to your instructor: fears, doubts, and questions can become the extra gear for your practice!

If you don't feel safe in the water, always try to follow this simple rule: avoid deep water and keep your feet on the ground (pool's floor, I mean)!

Partner up

We have seen it several times: sport, and in general, each of the activities presented in this book not only helps on a physical level but also and above all, on a mental and social level.

Under this last point, therefore, choosing a training partner is helpful and funny: you can perform the exercises by counting on one shoulder, you can encourage yourself and have fun in a sort of 'community rite.' It is liberating and full of meaning!

Water Equipment

After talking and giving a quick overview of the main physical activities in the water, here we focus on the leading equipment that you may need to perform these workouts in the best possible way and to fully benefit from the advantages deriving from these aquatic exercises. Here they come!

Swimming goggles

Some purists will argue that they don't need glasses, and while they're not required, it's something that will make you better.

Still, there are two fundamental reasons why you should always wear goggles in the pool:

- First, you need to have a good field of vision to swim safely among other swimmers and correctly judge the distance between you and the wall;
- Second, they will protect your eyes from redness and irritation. Although eye redness passes relatively quickly after getting out of the pool, it is much better to avoid it for health and hygiene reasons.

Swimming cap

Swim caps are worn for various reasons, and keeping hair off your face while swimming is one of them. The other is to protect you from the corrosive effects of chemicals used in swimming pools.

Of course, there are situations where you would prefer not to wear a hat. Some pools are very hot, so wearing a cap is most uncomfortable.

Two swimming caps are commonly used in training: silicone and latex.

Silicone is more durable, usually more comfortable, slightly more expensive, and will leave your head a bit warmer.

Latex caps are cheap, not as durable, but more breathable than silicone caps.

Swimming shoes

Using these shoes can come in handy if you have problems with your balance. You can buy them at most well-stocked supermarkets or sporting goods stores. Choose a model that offers a good ground grip and ensure it is comfortable.

The premium feature is a treaded outsole, which means they offer good grip on the pool floor.

Training swimsuit

A training suit is one of the beginner swimming accessories that will make you improve.

When choosing a workout suit, make sure it's comfortable and gives you a free range of motion in your hips. Please select the appropriate size so they are not loose or too tight.

Today, perhaps the most common choice is the so-called 'jammers'; they are suits just above the knee. They are able not to create resistance in the water and are also very comfortable. You can also choose other cuts, such as briefs.

Earplugs
This can also fall into the mandatory category for swimmers who need to wear earplugs. Wearing them is necessary to prevent water from entering the ear canals, which can lead to infection. Earaches are, without a doubt, the worst.
Earplugs can sometimes help you feel better in the water. Get plugs if you can't stand a bit of water around the ear area. Cone-shaped plugs are best, but special plastic plugs can be shaped like your ear.

Swimming board

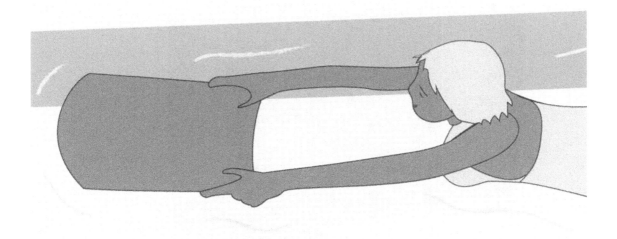

This is one of the essential - and most common - swimming accessories for beginners that will make you improve. It is a teaching and performance enhancer as it can help you improve your leg shape and balance in the water.

Pull buoy

The pull buoy is a really great training tool. It is a foaming aid with a unique 'eight' shape. You can place it between the knees, thighs, or ankles. It allows the training of the arms and raises the legs. Excellent help to exercise the rotation of the body as well.

For beginners, pull buoys can help with body alignment and promote positive posture while swimming. The pull buoyancy helps raise your lower body, so you are aligned in the water.

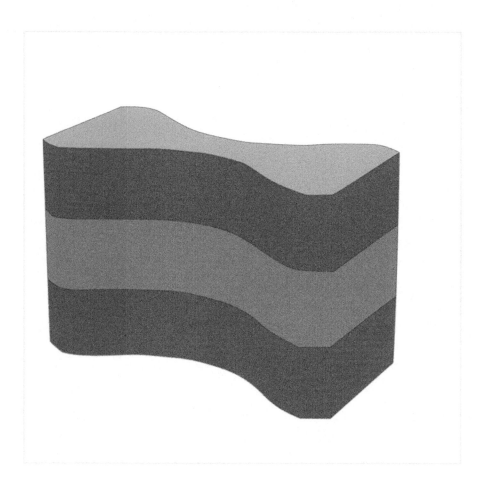

Chapter 5
18 Must-Know Exercises

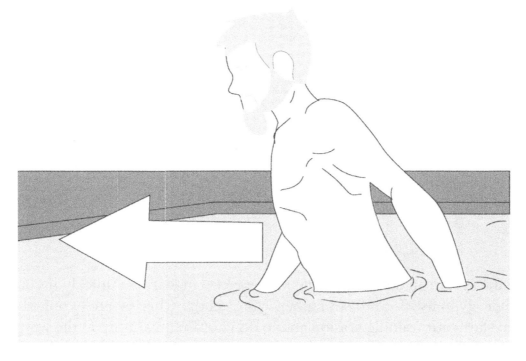

Water is much denser than air and offers more excellent resistance. This is why exercise in the water requires more effort than the same exercise on land and allows you to strengthen the muscles to a much greater extent.

It also helps burn more calories, which can aid in weight loss.

To perform this exercise, therefore, just take a walk at your pace in the pool. For added safety, you can find a workmate or use the edges as support to ensure the balance and protection you need.

AQUA JOGGING

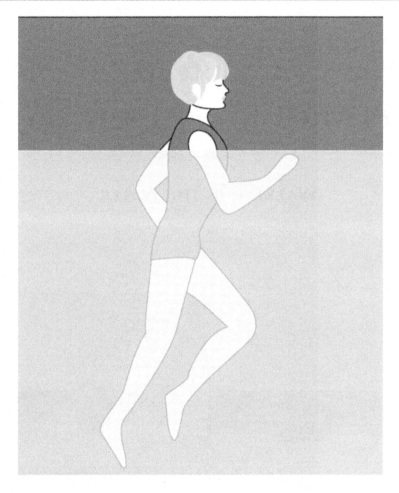

Running on the spot or in the water is the first exercise in learning quickly if you want to practice water gymnastics and strengthen your body. This is an excellent type of movement to start your training session and to do your first warm-up in the water.

You need to start slowly at the pace of a walk and then increase your pace. You will find yourself running in place gradually, keeping the pace for about two minutes.

When warming up with running in place, keeping your abdomen constantly tight is vital. The support on the bottom of the pool must be stable.

Moreover, for your balance, it is advisable to lean on the pool's edge. For those who want more support, it is advisable to wear special shoes for aqua aerobics, which guarantee more outstanding grip on the seabed.

FORWARD LUNGES

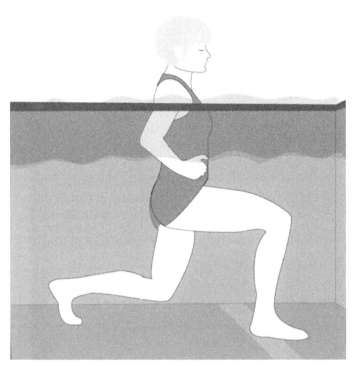

For these exercises, it is advisable to position yourself in an area of the pool where the water reaches just above the waist. It is then necessary to keep the torso very straight and put the hands on the hips.

Bring your right leg forward and press on the bottom of the pool with your foot.

After a few seconds, you can return to the starting position and lunge with the left. It is essential to continue alternating legs until the end of the session.

SIDE LUNGES

For this exercise, it is necessary to position yourself in the water that is not too high, with your legs slightly open, keeping your torso erect and your arms at your sides, with your hands with your palms open.

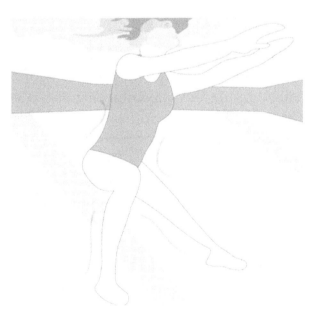

The movement consists in letting oneself slide first on one side and then on the other along the thighs, trying to maintain the torso straight as much as possible.

As in many exercises of this type, the trunk and neck must always remain straight.

FLUTTER KIKS

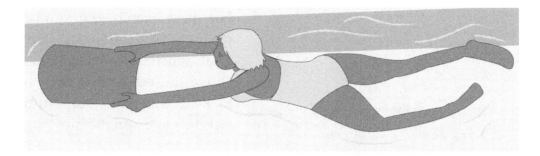

The technical support for training the legs is the classic swimming board. Using the tablet allows you to isolate the lower part of the body and concentrate training exclusively on the kick technique.

The board, when used well, is made to support the swimmer's buoyancy and maintain the best position in the water.

The tablet must be gripped on both sides on its upper part so that you can also place the elbows on it. If the head is raised during leg training with the tablet, you can also work in part on the abdominal wall muscles.

In addition to the board, you can also use fins or half fins.

FRONT LEG KICK

Bring the stretched leg forward until the tip of the foot emerges from the water: do this movement giving the maximum leg speed, and bring it back to the starting position, trying to maintain the rhythm.

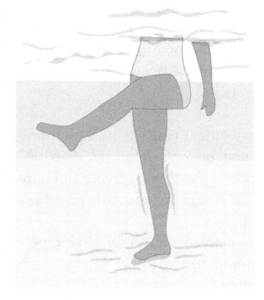

The resistance that water opposes when you simulate kicks will have a profound rejuvenate effect on your legs.

Take three series of 10 kicks in the water per leg, resting 30 seconds between one series and the next.

BACK LEG KICK

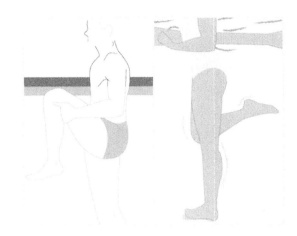

Tablet forward, horizontal underwater, arms supported, and torso flexed. The right leg is on the bottom; the left is bent at the chest.

Forcefully extend the leg back until it touches the bottom with the toe. Repeat 20 times on both legs.

PECTORAL PULL

Legs apart and abdominals contracted, hold two boards and hold them vertically underwater.

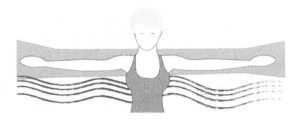

Forcefully close your arms by bringing the waves together.

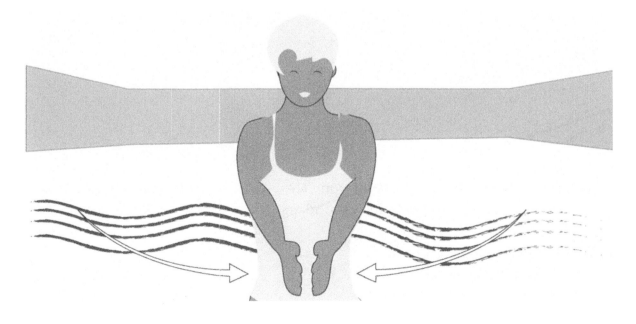

JUMP ON THE WATER

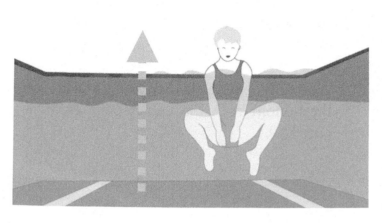

Go where the water reaches your shoulders and jump with your legs, bringing your knees to your chest.

This exercise will tone not only your legs but also your glutes!

The idea is to make as many jumps as you can within 30 seconds.

WATER SQUAT

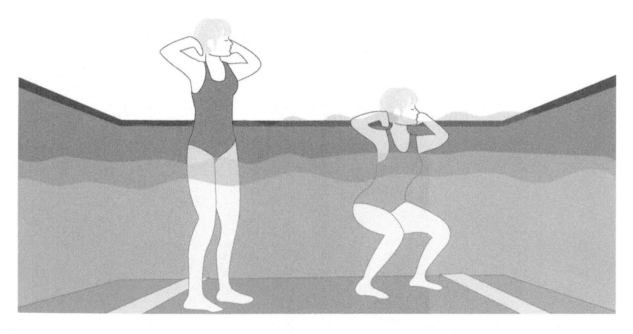

Move your pelvis back slowly and bend your legs, always moving slowly downwards. Whenever your thighs are parallel to the ground, stop and keep your back straight.

Don't take your heels off the ground.
Repeat the squats for 30 seconds for three sets.

SIDE LEG LIFT

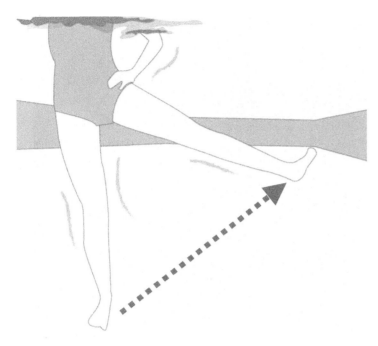

This type of exercise mainly helps to fight cellulite since the resistance of the water makes the muscles work and tones them.

To perform them, it is necessary to position yourself in front of the edge of the pool and raise your legs sideways about 30 times.

Subsequently, you can put your back to the edge and start lifting your legs forward, as the previous exercise with kicks.

In these sessions, however, it is necessary to keep the straight leg in place for a few seconds before returning to lower it. The longer you maintain the position, the more you train your muscles.

BICYCLE LEG LIFT

Without touching the bottom, keep the upright position and move your feet and legs as if you were on a bicycle.

Continue for almost 2 minutes. Simple and effective... just like riding a bicycle!

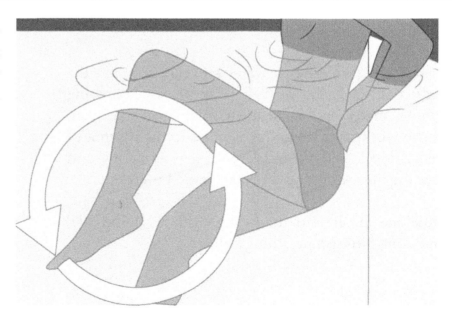

LEG SWINGS

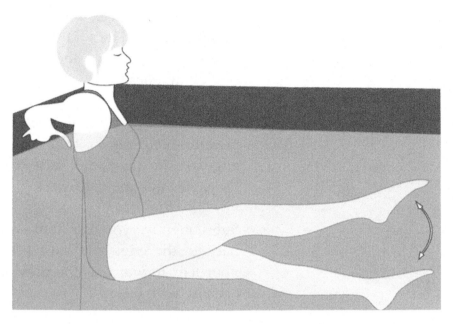

To perform this exercise, it is necessary to float on the back and flap the legs for a few minutes.

If you do not know how to swim well, it is advisable to perform the scissoring while remaining attached to the edge of the pool.

WATER ARM PUNCH

Just like boxing in all respects but practiced in the water: kicks and punches are slowed down by the resistance it opposes to your blows, but this is precisely what makes the muscle work and results in very effective toning.

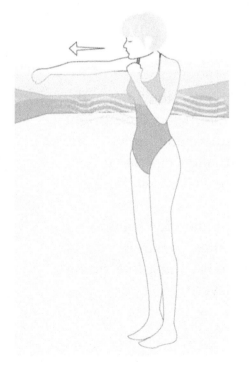

Furthermore, working in water serves to contain the production of lactic acid in the phases following training, increases the cardiovascular level thanks to intense work (which also takes place to the rhythm of music), develops the muscles of the legs and arms, and tones the muscles of the core (abs, back, buttocks).

Stand and push into the water with a closed fist, simulating hitting a punching ball.

STANDING KNEE LIFT

To perform this exercise, you must learn to float (or use the kick board).

Lying in the water, bring your knees to your chest and swim to maintain the balance.

Repeat from the beginning for ten pushes.

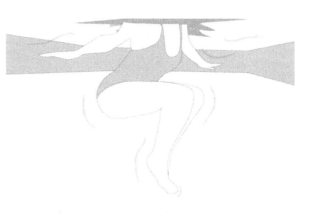

WATER TAXI

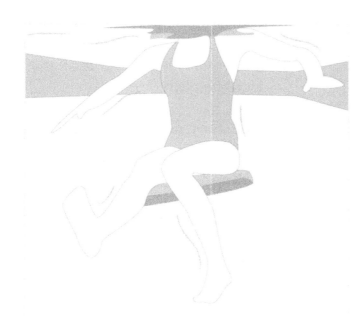

Sit on the kick board and, with your arms in front of you, sweep them out to the sides as if you're doing breaststroke, traveling across the pool for 30 seconds.

Use the strength in your arms to move around.

For the next 30 seconds, switch your stroke, going in the opposite direction, bringing your arms together in front of your body with your palms facing in.

STANDING WATER PUSH-UPS

This one is performed if you do not have any particular back pain or joint issue.

To start, stand along the side of the pool. Place your hands on the edge, wider than shoulder-width apart.

Bend your arms, and then lean in toward the wall. Push yourself back out and repeat this exercise slowly until your arms feel tired.

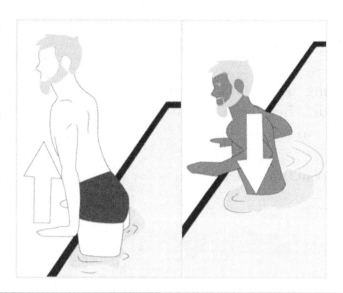

EGGBEATER KICK

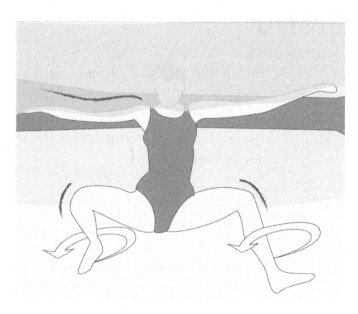

The eggbeater kick requires the legs to move in opposite directions.

First of all, find yourself a standard "water chair." Sit on the edge of it and let your legs hang, bent at a 90-degree angle.

Then start moving with your right leg. Just move it circularly clockwise or counterclockwise.

Once you are comfortable with that movement, use your left leg and continue in a clockwise position.

Do one leg at a time, circularly moving your legs until you are feeling ok with that.

At all times, there's gonna be a leg going in and another leg going out.

Chapter 6
Water Aerobics Circuits for Seniors

These are the best workouts for seniors that will enhance body fitness, rehabilitations, strength training and others.

'LOW PROFILE' CIRCUIT

As we saw earlier, there are many activities proposed in the pool, but it is not mandatory to enroll in one of these courses! Of course, it is always recommended to have an instructor who guides and advises you, but you can also do your exercises independently if you know how to do them.

Below you will find an example of a circuit to adapt to your initial training state. Each exercise tones and works on a specific part of the body, without too many thoughts on 'perfection' or execution. Simply trying and being active, focusing on a single muscle group at a time, has its effects. And this is more true in the water!

The ideal would be to repeat it 2 or 3 times in a row, with 1 minute of consistently walking in the water, between one series and the next. You should repeat each exercise 15 times, and between one activity and another, it is best to allow yourself a break of at least 20 seconds.

WARM-UP

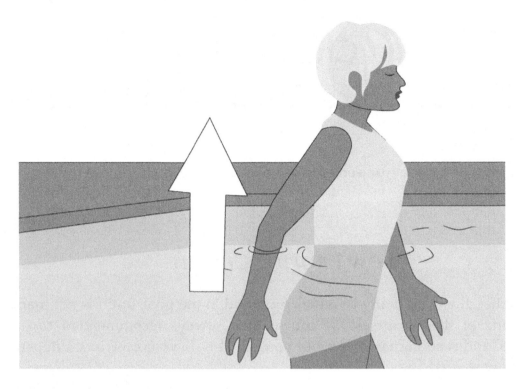

Start with a 5-minute walk in the water.

PECTORALS

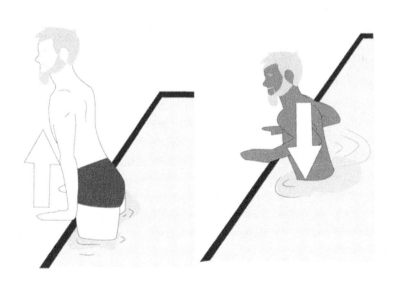

In the water up to the shoulders, feet as far apart as the pelvis.

Raise your arms outstretched in line with your shoulders while your elbows remain flexed at 90 ° flush with the water.

As you exhale, close your arms towards your torso, immerse them entirely and, inhale, return to the starting position.

261

ABDOMINALS

Lie on your stomach in the water, getting used to a board if n e c e s s a r y. Extend your arms forward, keeping your elbows slightly bent and your legs back.

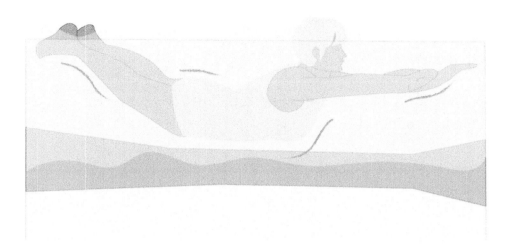

Lift your chest off the ground by using your lower back muscles. Keep your neck and arms aligned with your spine. Be very careful when doing this exercise.

Don't lift your chest and legs at the same time - if you did, you would be exerting extreme effort with the back discs. Likewise, do not raise your head more than 20cm.

Breathing in, put your feet back on the bottom, and return to the starting position.

THIGHS

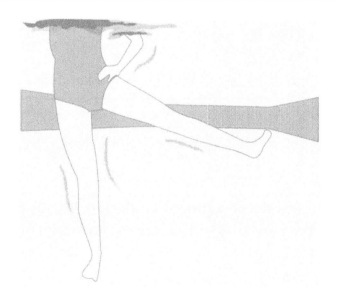

Arms outstretched, exhale side kick by lifting the leg and keeping the knee slightly bent as you push the arms down.

To be performed alternating the leg.

TWIST AND HIPS

With legs and arms spread at the same height, rotate only the torso to the right and then to the left.

Keep your head firm and straight, with the gaze aimed straight ahead.

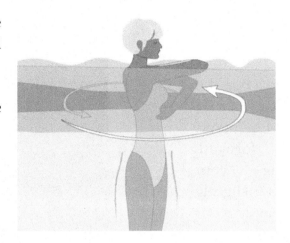

BUTTOCKS

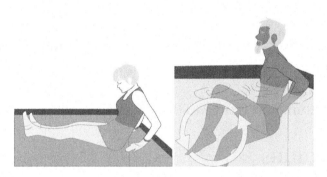

Arms wide, not in tension.

Bringing your knees towards your chin and stretching them out in front of you simulates a pedal stroke as if you were sitting on an exercise bike.

FINAL STRETCH

You can do some stretching exercises in the water or relax with breaststroke style... or free style!

This is an example of a circuit for water aerobics and gymnastics with low-impact on your body.

I do not recommend starting physical activity before consulting your doctor. Also, if you are more inexperienced, it is always better to sign up for a course and rely on a professional to start your practice.

TONING CIRCUIT

Water aerobic training requires moderate and prolonged effort over time. Among the main advantages of water aerobics, we remember that it aims to define the muscles, improve the cardiovascular system and lose weight, ease worries and find a fun dimension from a psychological point of view. It looks similar to other sports like water aerobics or aquafitness, right?

The best way to achieve this form of physical and mental well-being is to gradually approach aerobic training through these simple water aerobics exercises.

JOGGING ON THE SPOT

The run on the spot in the pool starts with slow movements and results in a high knee run at a slightly more intense pace.

Aerobic exercise must be accompanied by the movement of the arms in the frontal plane or the sagittal plane, depending on the rhythm imposed by the lower limbs.

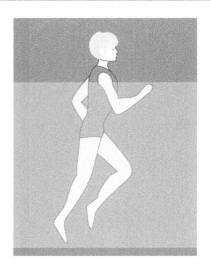

SCISSORING IN PLACE

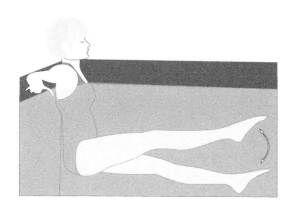

Scissoring in place requires standing with support on the bottom and proceeding with simultaneous movements of all limbs along the sagittal plane.

Stand with your back straight, move your legs and arms and let your body weight fall on the forward leg, all without moving your torso.

ELEVATOR

The curious name hides a simple and, at the same time, effective movement from the aerobic point of view.

It is enough to stand up straight, spread your legs shoulder-width apart and plant your feet on the bottom before coming down with your torso while keeping your back straight.

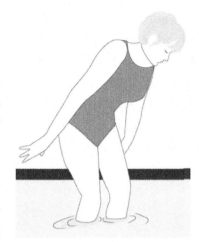

The essential thing in this exercise is not to work the abdominals but to concentrate everything on the buttocks and accompany the movement using the arms to find balance.

JUMP IN COLLECTION

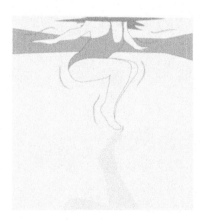

Collection jumps involve a jump that ends by bringing the knees to the chest and opening the arms both sides.

You can strengthen aerobic work simply by contracting the abdominal muscles, closing the shoulders 'egg', and exhaling in the closing phase before returning to the starting position.

TWISTS

The twist in the water requires a square body position with bent legs, a movement of the water with the hands, and a rotation of the torso on the horizontal axis.

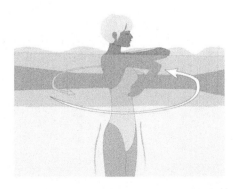

OPENING AND CLOSING OF THE UPPER LIMBS

All that needs to be done to perform the exercise is to stand on the ground with legs apart at the same width as the shoulders, arms open under the surface of the water, and forearms in extension.

Begin to open and close the outstretched arms with palms facing towards the outside.

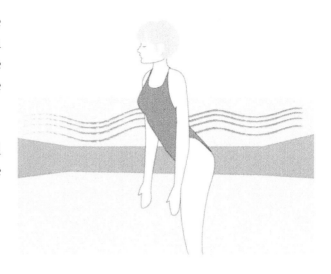

ENERGIZING CIRCUIT

WARM-UP: RUNNING ON THE SPOT

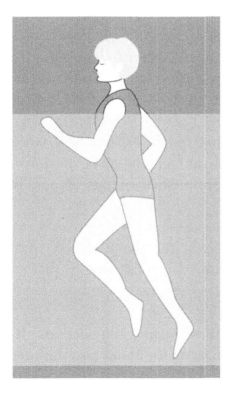

Running on the spot is the first exercise in learning quickly if you want to practice water gymnastics and strengthen your body. This is an excellent type of movement to start your training session and to do your first warm-up in the water. You need to start slowly at the pace of a walk and then increase your pace. You will find yourself running in place gradually, keeping the pace for about two minutes.

When warming up with running in place, keeping your abdomen constantly tight is vital. The support on the bottom of the pool must be stable. Moreover, for your balance, it is advisable to lean on the pool's edge. For those who want more support, it is advisable to wear special shoes for aqua aerobics, which guarantee more outstanding grip on the seabed.

HIGH KNEES

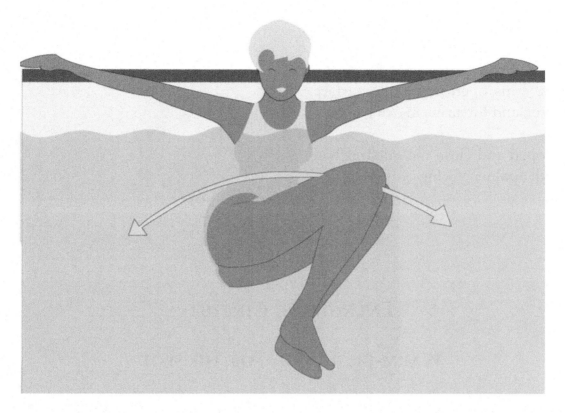

Once you prepare your cardiovascular system with running on the spot, it's time to tackle the second water gymnastics exercise, running with high knees. Also used as a warm-up, this exercise is the natural continuation of the first, with a slight increase in the level of effort required. However, this is not a complicated athletic gesture, even if it requires a particular strength if performed at high intensity.

Proceeding step by step means not necessary to push that much, especially if we are beginners and need to get back in shape. Therefore, the movement to be performed requires that during the race (always in place), the knees are pushed as high as possible, towards the chest, and alternately.

Here too, the abdomen must remain constantly contracted for the duration of the exercise, which develops in two phases. In the first phase, you must run in place by pushing your knees as high as possible for twenty seconds.

The second moment, on the other hand, consists of a pause lasting ten seconds. It is enough to repeat the exercise for three or four sets, going to work for about two minutes.

CONTROLLED OSCILLATIONS

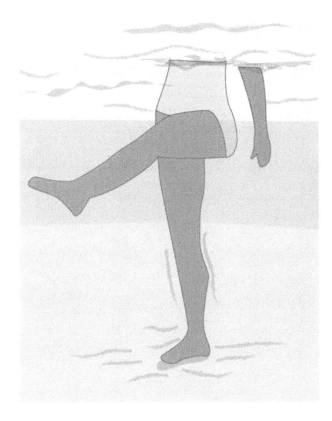

After completing the first warm-up exercises, we are already beginning to feel the benefits, especially in the legs, with water gymnastics that awaken circulation and regain vitality and the muscles that wake up from a long lethargy. We then insist on the legs, going to train them with a series of controlled swings.

You can also perform the oscillations with a small gym dumbbell in hand to balance the body's weight during the movements, increasing balance and toning the arms simultaneously.

You have to remain standing on one leg, leaning on the edge of the pool with the corresponding hand. The other leg is lifted, keeping the foot in a hammer position.

At this point, it is sufficient to carry out a rotational movement of the hip with the leg well stretched, performing twenty oscillations with one leg, and then the other.

With this exercise, the buttocks, the lower abdominals, and the lateral abdominals are toned up, the neck muscles are strengthened - and the arms if you use the dumbbells. In this case, you must keep the handlebar in your hand, at head height, with your arm bent at ninety degrees.

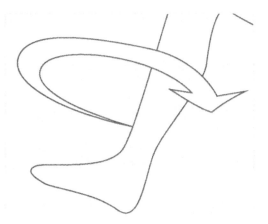

Repeat the exercise with the opposite part of the body at the change of leg.

JUMPING JACK

The subsequent water gymnastics exercise consists of a series of hops with the body that must coordinate the movements of the arms and legs. You have to position yourself away from the edge because you need to move your arms in this case, and it is essential to make sure you have enough space available.

We start standing, with the torso very straight and the spine aligned with the neck, knees, and feet, well stable on the bottom of the pool.

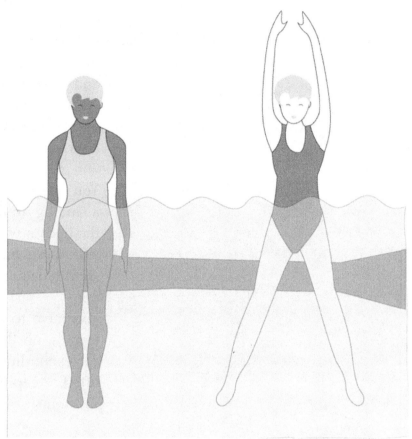

From this position, you start by opening and closing both the arms and the legs simultaneously, in such a way as to perform small jumps on the spot. With the palms of the hands, you have to make alternating thrusts, once inwards and the next time outwards.

The complete movement (therefore an opening and a closing) must be performed for ten repetitions, then for another twenty, in which ten to push firmly towards the outside, and the last ten with a firm push towards the inside.

To help yourself in the pushes to be carried out with the hands, it is helpful to help yourself with the specific water aerobics dumbbells if you want to increase the effort of the arms. These tools are also very useful in coordinating movement, to perform the exercise in a more fluid way and with a more symmetrical action of the whole body.

CIRCLING THE LEGS

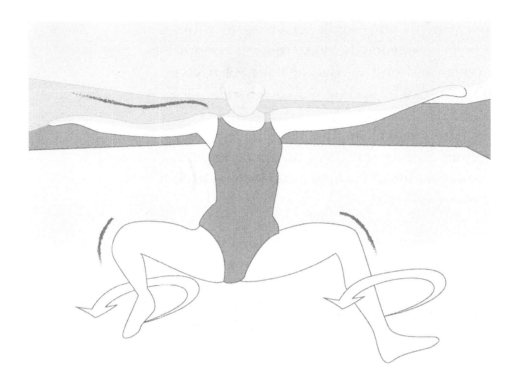

After the jumping jacks, once we have recovered our breath by taking a break of about 60 seconds, we proceed with the circling of the legs. This exercise primarily tones your legs and abs and helps improve balance even after you get out of the pool.

The starting position is the classic one, standing away from the poolside.

Keeping the left leg firmly, you begin to move the right leg with lateral rotational movements. The movement must first be performed with the foot near the bottom and then gradually raise the leg higher and higher. Keeping the foot in the classic hammer position and the leg rigid, it is thus necessary to perform five rotations of the limb clockwise and five counterclockwise.

To help balance, the arm opposite the moving leg performs the same movements but in the opposite direction to support itself through the thrust of the water to maintain the correct position.

Once you have finished the ten repetitions, you immediately move on to training the other leg, completely reversing the exercise on the other side without taking rest breaks.

BULL MOVEMENT

The Bull Movement is the sixth exercise to train comfortably at home or outside the pool. You can perform it both in the center and on the edge of the pool if you want to find more balance by leaning with one hand.

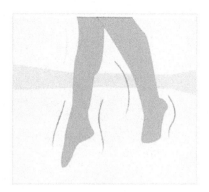

The starting position is again standing, with the legs very stable at the bottom of the pool. Then move one leg at a time, mimicking the motion of the angry bull kicking back before running towards its prey.

One leg, therefore, remains stationary while the other performs a fast flexion (how fast you have to decide based on your level of training) back, bending the knee with the heel that goes towards the buttocks.

The exercise effectively trains the quadriceps, hamstring, and glutes above all, with benefits also for the whole upper and lower abdominal belt and, to a lesser extent, the oblique abdominal compartment.

ABDOMINAL BAND

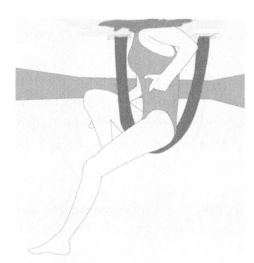

The abdominal band is also fun because it is performed with the help of the classic colored water aerobics float tube. The tube must be placed immediately under the armpits or between the legs and must emerge from the water.

The starting position is seated, with the feet held in a hammer and the torso bent at ninety degrees concerning the legs. These must initially be extended well, then you start by opening and closing the limbs twenty times without pause.

It is possible to increase the level of effort by increasing the number of repetitions because the floating tube helps a lot to decrease the thrust, making the exercise accessible to anyone.

LIFT AND STRETCH

The starting position is the same as in the previous practice, with one arm resting on the edge of the pool.

The movement changes because you have to flex your knee, until you reach your chest. During the whole movement, the feet must be stretched well, with the toes in constant extension.

Then extend the leg forward, slowly return to the starting position. The exercise must be repeated twenty times, alternating the legs, again without pausing.

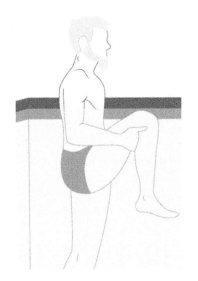

HIGH-KNEES TWIST

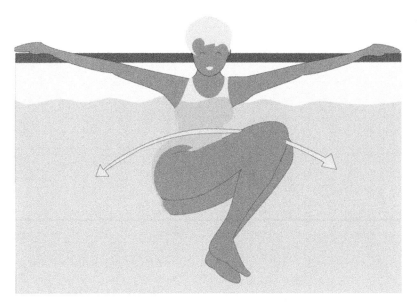

This exercise of water aerobics closes the series of abdominals in the water and engages the entire sideband. It is called Twist and should also be performed here, resting on the pool's edge or using the aqua aerobics tube.

The starting position is the same as in the previous exercise, but the movement, in this case, is lateral, rotating the legs to the left and then to the right twenty times.

BOOK 6:
ALL-IN WORKOUTS AND EXERCISES FOR SENIORS

Chapter 1
Your Time, Your Rules

Hey you ... I am thrilled that we have come together with the juicy part of the whole book: our beloved workouts!

Yeah: because now that you know what the best exercises, routines, and circuits you want to do to strengthen your posture, flexibility, core, and balance and become more physically-mentally-emotionally powerful are... it's time to build your optimal training time day by day.

By 'optimal training,' we mean the best ratio between training intensity and duration, correct training frequency, and use of the most suitable exercises based on individual physical and postural characteristics, especially at 50-60 years old and more. So, let's dig in.

Let's start by talking about the correct training duration/intensity ratio: the intensity must always be privileged concerning the duration of the single training session since, after about 50 minutes from the beginning of the training, there is a progressive increase in the release of some hormones, including cortisol. This hormone tends to create further protein lysis, which is counterproductive, especially if you seek to improve muscle tone.

If you perform your training seriously, then, after 35-40 minutes, the muscle fibers will be exhausted. Still, you will have already done your vital work of love for yourself.

So: what's the ideal weekly frequency for training? The answer to that doubt is not as simple as it seems: compared to the canonical three weekly sessions, in fact, very often, it is possible to obtain excellent results already with two weekly sessions. The muscle, in fact, 'grows' during rest: that's why, if we do not give the body time to recover both at a muscular and mental level, we risk going into 'overtraining.' And that phase of overtraining can lead to poor (or even counterproductive) results, especially within our minds.

To understand if it is better to train 2, 3, or 4 times a week, therefore, it is necessary to perfectly know our bodies and our recovery skills, which depend on various factors. These can include:

• psycho-emotional-mental characteristics of the person;

- quality and quantity of food ingested;
- type of work done;
- stress levels.

If someone works ten hours a day, eats little, and is stressed due to family and/or relationship problems, they will need to reduce training administration (in some cases, even once a week is sufficient), at least until some variants - such as nutrition and stress - have not improved.

As regards the use of the most suitable exercises, for example, a careful evaluation of the individual characteristics is necessary, both from a musculoskeletal and postural point of view, to identify which muscles that need to be toned and which are stretched without running into injuries, muscle pains, or problems of body asymmetries.

Furthermore, there are no right and wrong exercises, but there is the person who, as such, has a concrete muscle reality on which it is necessary to work specifically to obtain the best result with the lower risk involved.

One question now arises spontaneously: if I want to improve my body in its entirety, but I have limitations that do not recommend performing some exercises aimed at toning the group muscle mentioned above, how can I develop all this?

For example, you want to work on muscle rebalancing in the first periods (let's say about 2-3 months), with professional support, and, after having achieved this, you can begin to use exercises on those muscle groups that were initially only stretching work was done.

In short, the classic and still in vogue in many gyms Monday card: chest-biceps, Wednesday: back-triceps, Friday: shoulders-legs-abdomen, cannot work anymore and definitely for everyone!

Understanding individual needs also mean stopping to reflect on what you need to improve your physical condition, getting out of the now-gone concept that 'more is better.

This is why, therefore, this book begins with the Statement 'My Time, my Rules': you can start slowly, understand how your body works thanks to the help of the exercises, and choose, from time to time, how much time you want to devote to your training.

Without overdoing it, without the anxiety of the performance, but with the desire to grow both physically and spiritually ... and not only at the age level!

If you are here, I am sure it is because your search for physical well-being has made you understand how fundamental it is to rebuild that relationship with ourselves that our society requires us to ignore.

Well: now you can claim it with pride!

These workouts, therefore, are full-body jobs that are based on the time available to the practitioner: if you are looking for specific flows to work on certain parts of the body or to

restore balance following pain, injuries, etc., you can refer to the previous books and also to Book 7, where we will deal with the workouts dedicated to your Wellness!
Good work!

Chapter 2
Your Training Plan

Physical activity - I have repeated several times - is the pillar of our day that supports health, vigor, and mood and gives a harmonious body.

So, how much, which one, and how to choose it?

Exercise is known to be healthy for young and old alike; unfortunately, our day is marked by numerous commitments. Between daily activities and family, it is not easy to find time to do physical activity. Still, above all, for many, it is not a priority. For it to become, however, you must reinforce motivation.

There are at least three reasons that should prompt us to exercise regularly, especially as we get older:

• a study published in April 2015 based on a sample of over 300,000 people from 10 different countries confirms that physical activity reduces the risk of mortality for all, both thin and obese, males and females, while the risk increases for those who do minor or moderate activity and for sedentary people;

• structured and adequate physical exercise shapes the body, makes it more agile, protects it more from fractures, and makes it more harmonious and robust;

• a physical activity carried out habitually has positive effects on our nervous and hormonal systems. It also facilitates learning and mindfulness, improving mood and fighting depression.

The reduction in mortality risk confirms what many studies have already shown: physical activity gives well-being and helps prevent even major diseases, consequently 'prolongs life.'

But what is fundamental is the quantity and intensity with which it is practiced, and each person must identify their limits to ensure that it is neither too much nor too little.

In general, medical guidelines for seniors and adults recommend at least 150 minutes a week of moderate-intensity aerobic physical activity to prevent weight gain and a balanced diet. And that works if practiced for at least ten consecutive minutes (without stopping).

Moreover, 300 minutes a week is optimal for anyone who wants to reduce disease and mortality risk.

What is the physical activity recommended? Optimal physical activity is that which engages both the cardiovascular, respiratory, and musculoskeletal systems without causing damage to joints and bones, e.g .:
• Perform a moderate intensity alternating with vigorous aerobic workout for a minimum duration of 40-50 minutes without breaks 4 or 6 times a week. Walking, running, cycling, swimming, and dancing are terrific;
• Perform an anaerobic muscle strengthening workout 2-4 times a week with increasing repetitions. Bodyweight exercises, with weights or machines, or without them.

How to structure your training

Constant workouts over time, different on alternate days, with inactive periods not exceeding 48 hours, even carried out on the same day, for example, on Sunday, one hour in the morning and one in the afternoon or a one or 2-hour match, etc.
Walking also gives good results to young and old; walking has a lot of potential. It can be practiced at moderate intensity (3 or 4 km/hour) and vigorous (5-6 km/hour). You can walk on mixed routes for long periods, even a few hours.
Dancing can be considered an excellent weekly aerobic exercise, especially if the time spent is added to other activities; for example: walking three times a week for a total of 180 minutes and dancing for 120 becomes a 300-minute workout, as long as the dance is done with a certain intensity, not a slow one.
You may also need an activity that 'burns' the stored fats while maintaining training over time. In fact, for the first 10-15 minutes, our body consumes the 'ready sugars' introduced with food, and it is only in the following minutes that it will begin to take energy from the 'fats' we have accumulated; on average, after 20 minutes you begin to consume both fats and sugars, continuing the workout you will come to consume less and less sugar and more fats until you only consume fat, which on average occurs after about an hour of activity.

Physical activity as a part of our day

Just as our eating day is structured with breakfast, lunch, dinner, and two snacks, so should the training program be carried out every day.

Let's take a concrete example of the protocol that a typical 50-70-year-old person of average weight should follow:

• 10-15 minutes of chair yoga or light gymnastics every morning;
• every Monday, Wednesday, Friday, and Sunday, at any time, 30-40 minutes of aerobic workout, including 2 minutes of vigorous intensity every 10 minutes of moderate;
• every Tuesday, Thursday, and Saturday, at any time, 30 minutes of anaerobic exercise.

It's a Matter of Lifestyle

Physical activity is a crucial component of the lifestyle of people who want to gain health and balanced and proper nutrition.

Of course, it is not mandatory to join the gym to carry out physical activity. All you need are comfortable shoes, a little initiative, and a lot of consistency. You can walk at a good pace, run, ride a bicycle, climb stairs, and do bodyweight exercises that still use the muscles of both the upper and lower limbs and the abdominals. Simple activities you can do outdoors or at home.

Even those who lead a hectic life and never seem to have time for themselves can choose to exercise in one of these three moments; just keep in mind that for each of these, there are rules and tips to remember.

Awakening Training

Early in the morning, before starting the day, a little free body gymnastics (muscle awakening), chair yoga routines, or stretching (only for those who are able to) can be instrumental in loosening the joints that have remained still during the night. When you do your workout, before starting your day, remember that it is necessary to reactivate the cardio-circulatory and respiratory system, so move gently and gradually for about half an hour to avoid getting too tired and consuming too much energy that will be used for the rest of the day.

Complete your morning awakening with a light and happy breakfast.

Afternoon 'Me Time' Training

If you want to train during the afternoon, it is best to engage in anaerobic exercises without exaggerating so as not to go back to work with sore muscles. Although aerobic muscle strengthening certainly involves a lower calorie consumption than an aerobic workout, it is advisable to have an afternoon snack to avoid arriving too hungry for dinner.

Before Bed Training

If you choose this time to train, do it with awareness and happiness: stretching routines, bedtime yoga on the mat or on the bed, or even meditation are ideal. You will not consume the same calories as your workouts out in the open, but you will prepare the perfect space to sleep soundly and wake up with a high and happy spirit.

Chapter 3
Tips and Tricks

- Before undertaking any type of exercise (within these books as well), it is best to undergo a medical-sports examination.

- Practice aerobic activity initially with low intensity and gradually increase for optimal fat burning, alternating moments of more vigorous exercise.

- Provide for small sessions interspersed with short breaks, 30/60 seconds, especially in the first approaches to physical activity.

- In the summertime, avoid exercising during the hottest hours of the day or in too humid or cold environments in winter.

- Remember to drink at least 8-ounce standard glasses (2 liters of water per day) and during workouts, make sure you drink small amounts frequently to stay hydrated. It is essential to hydrate properly to replenish both fluids and mineral salts that are lost with sweating. In particular, this advice is helpful for those who practice outdoor sports, exposed to the sun.

- Choose the right equipment and clothing.

- Take advantage of every opportunity to move.

- Combine physical exercise with a balanced diet (see the next paragraph). Avoid exercising after consuming a large meal: if the body is very busy with digestion, it is less efficient in motor performance, and it's not comfortable (and you will notice that for sure). However, even avoiding physical activity on an empty stomach: muscles need energy to function correctly and essential proteins, especially branched-chain amino acids. The only exception is the 10-minute workout in the morning, which you can do even on an empty stomach. If anything, drink half a glass of water before starting.

Food Rules

- Follow a Mediterranean-type diet and respect the energy balance.

- Eat a light snack before exercising. Here are some examples: a snack based on bread, fruit, and Grana Padano, yogurt or milk and cereals, a small sandwich (about 50 g) stuffed with 30 g of bresaola, a salad with drained tuna and a little bread, after each small meal a fruit or a juice without sugar.

- Eat a regular breakfast. Those who have the opportunity to exercise in the morning can start with a cup of milk or yogurt accompanied by cereals or rusks or biscuits or bread with jam, plus fruit or juice.

- Prevent dehydration. During physical activity, you need to drink low-mineralized water (about two to three glasses); the stomach can dispose of 250 ml of water in less than 20 minutes.

- After the activity, if it is expected that a long time may pass before the next meal (lunch or dinner), it is good to have another light snack and fruit.

- If our goal is also to lose weight, we must not fast but adopt a balanced low-calorie diet calculated based on age, gender, body mass index (BMI), and medical advice.

Chapter 4
5-Minute Workout

Who: for you, when you feel tired or have a little time but want to train anyway.
What: with the chair (or standing Yoga asanas).
When: in the morning to start the day; in the afternoon.
Where: at home, on your terrace, on the beach (but not in the hot hours).
How: gently, without forcing the movements.
Why: set your intention for the practice: 'Today I choose this because ...'

Hold each pose for the specified time.

1. Mountain Pose - Sit firmly, eye closed. (20 seconds) (Pg. 30)
2. Squat + Tree Pose: Take a squat (20 seconds) and then take the Tree pose with a chair (hold for 10 seconds) - Right Side (Pg. 151 + Pg. 40)
3. Chair pose (Hold for 20 seconds) - 2 repetitions (Pg. 39)
4. Squat + Tree Pose: Take a squat (20 seconds) and then take the Tree pose with a chair (hold for -10 seconds) - Left Side (Pg. 151 + Pg. 40)
5. Chair pose (Hold for 10 seconds) (Pg. 39)
6. Warrior II on the chair (Hold for 15 seconds) - Right Side (Pg. 53)
7. Reverse Warrior II on the Chair (Hold for 10 seconds) - Right Side (Pg. 55)
8. Repeat n.6 and n.7 - (total: 25 seconds) - Left Side (Pg. 53 + Pg. 55)
9. Warrior I on the chair (Hold for 20 seconds) - Right Side (Pg. 52)
10. Warrior I on the chair (Hold for 20 seconds) - Left Side (Pg. 52)
11. Mountain Pose - Sit firmly, eye closed. (10 seconds) (Pg. 30)
12. Anjali Mudra Meditation (1 minute) (Pg. 32)

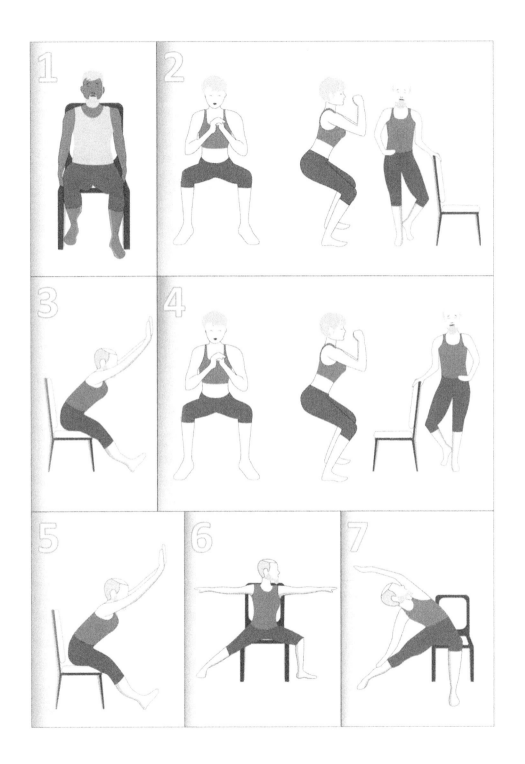

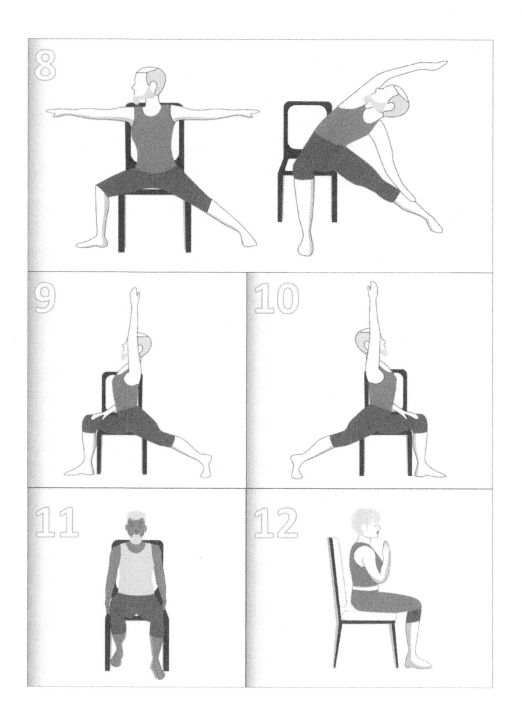

Chapter 5
10-Minute Workout

Who: for you, when you need a gentle practice, to be with yourself.
What: your bed, the mat.
When: in the morning to start the day; in the afternoon; before bed.
Where: at home, on your balcony, in the green.
How: gently, without forcing the movements.
Why: set your intention for the practice: 'Today I choose this because …'
Hold each pose for the specified time and perform the exercises carefully.

1. Savasana + Normally Breathing (1 minute + 15 seconds) (Pg. 43-45)
2. Hands circles (30 seconds)
3. Ankles circles laying or knees bent (1 minute)
4. Legs up and down (1 minute)
5. Legs on the side, alternate them (2 minutes and half) (Pg.190)

Carefully Transitioning in the seated position, legs crossed comfortably.

6. Tilt one side and the other (1 minute)
7. Arms up and press it back (1 minute)
8. Knees up and down (1 minute)

Carefully Transitioning into forward fold

9. Forward Fold Ragdoll (20 seconds) (Pg. 35-36)
10. Chair Pose (30 seconds) (Pg. 39)
11. Torso rotations (30 seconds)
12. Arms up and down (15 seconds)

Relax and say thank you!

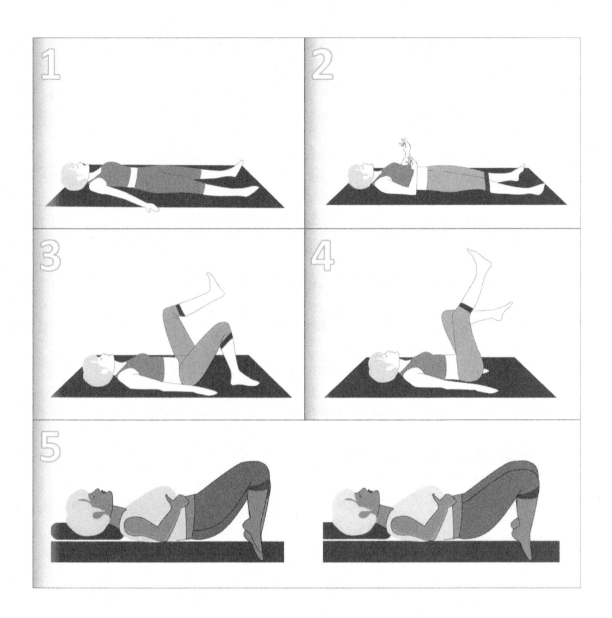

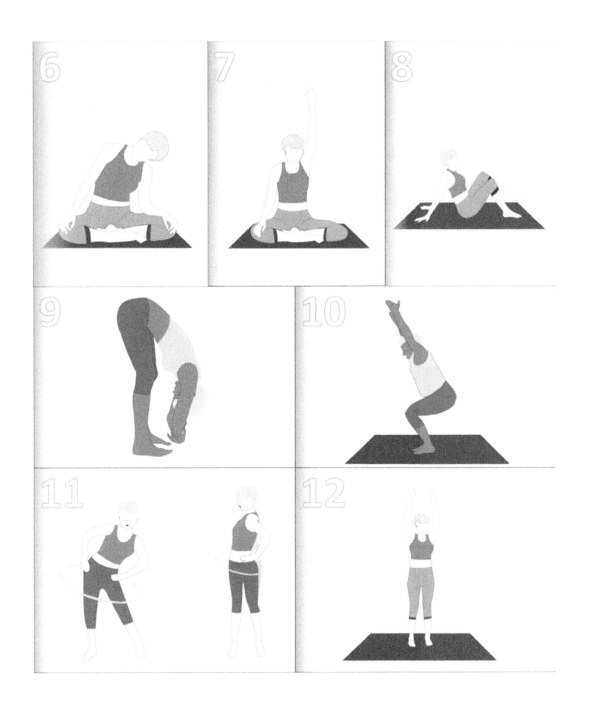

Chapter 6
16-Minute Workout

Who: for you, when you want to practice everyday.
What: your chair.
When: in the morning to start the day; in the afternoon; before bed.
Where: at home, on your balcony.
How: gently, without forcing the movements.
Why: set your intention for the practice: 'Today I choose this because ...'

Hold each pose for the specified time and perform the exercises carefully.

1. Mountain Pose - Sit firmly, eye closed. (40 seconds) (Pg. 30)
2. Breathing rest with Palms on Belly (1 minute) (Pg. 29)
3. Neck Releases: neck on the side (10 seconds), chin on the chest (10 seconds), neck right and left (10 seconds) (Pg. 23)
4. Hand gently pressing on the top of the head (30 seconds on each side)
5. Cat & Cow (30 seconds) (Pg. 31)
6. Right Side Bends (20 seconds) + Right Torsion (10 seconds) (Pg. 37)
7. Left Side Bends (20 seconds) + Left Torsion (10 seconds) (Pg. 37)
8. Half Sun Salutation - Hands up, forward fold, half forward fold, hands up (30 seconds) - 2 repetitions (Pg. 33; Pg. 35-36)
9. Forward fold Ragdoll (40 seconds) (Pg. 35-36)
10. Sit on the edge of the chair - Right Knee to chest (15 seconds) + Ankle roll (15 seconds) + Open the arms and hold (15 seconds) - Right Side (Pg. 34)
11. Sit on the edge of the chair - Right Knee to chest (15 seconds) + Ankle roll (15 seconds) + Open the arms and hold (15 seconds) - Left Side (Pg. 34)
12. Goddess pose (40 seconds) (Pg. 39)
13. Goddess pose Shoulder Release (20 seconds) - Right Side
14. Goddess pose Shoulder Release (20 seconds) - Left Side

15.Warrior II on the chair (Hold for 40 seconds) - Reverse Warrior on the Chair (Hold for 10 seconds) - Right Side + Extended Side Angle (20 seconds) - Right Side (Pg. 53; Pg. 55; Pg. 48)

16.Repeat n.15 sequence on the Left Side (Pg. 53; Pg. 55; Pg. 48)

17.Sit on the edge - Seated Pigeon Pose (1 minute) - Right Side (Pg. 56)

18.Sit on the edge - Seated Pigeon Pose (1 minute) - Left Side (Pg. 56)

19.Boat Pose (Hold for 40 seconds) (Pg. 49)

20.Savasana Relaxation (2 minutes) (Pg. 43-45)

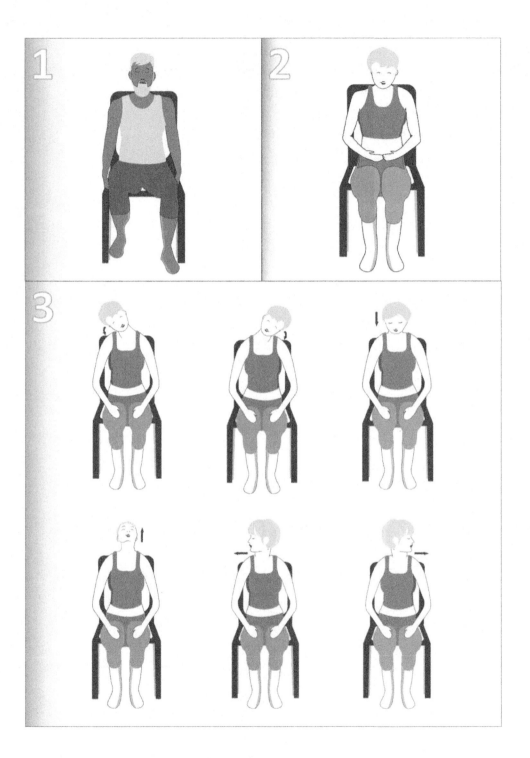

291

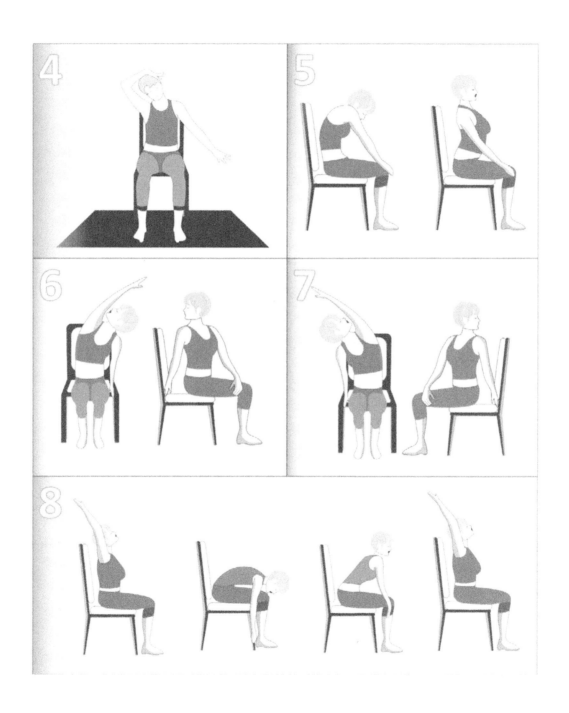

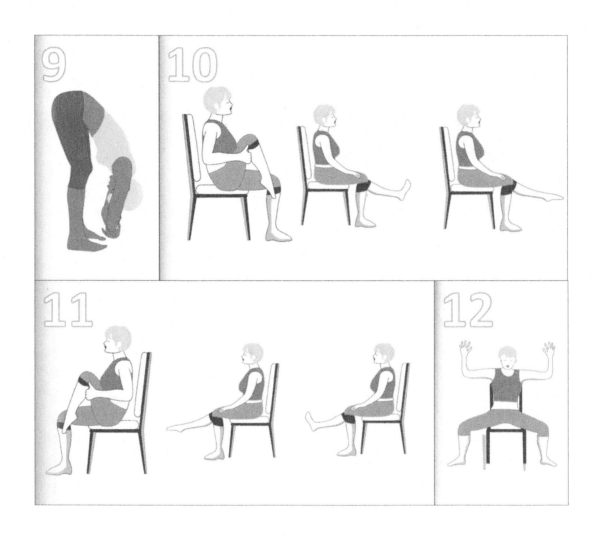

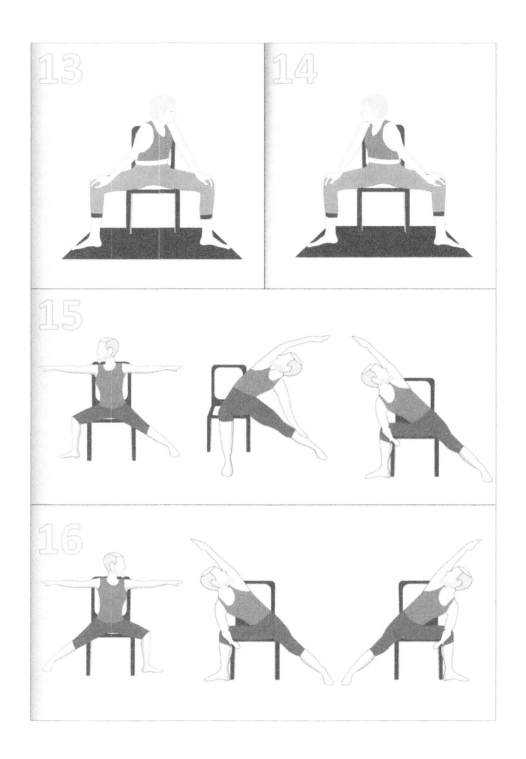

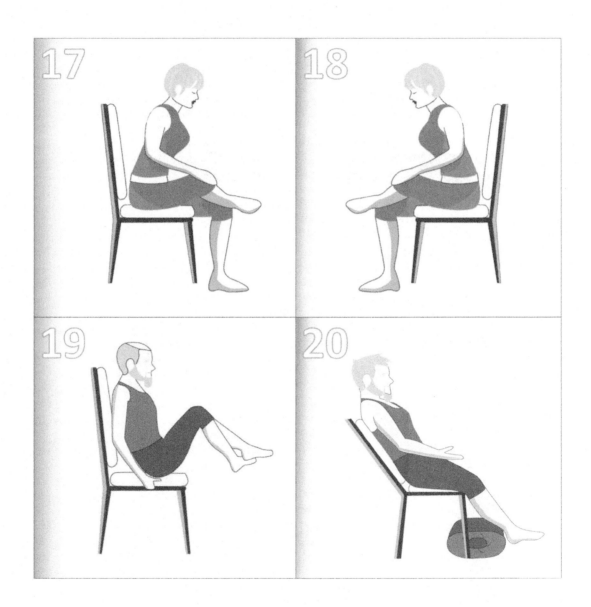

Chapter 7
30-Minute Workout

Who: for you, when you want to dig into the practise.
What: your chair.
When: in the morning to start the day; in the afternoon; before bed.
Where: at home, on your balcony.
How: gently, without forcing the movements.
Why: set your intention for the practice: 'Today I choose this because ...'

Hold each pose for the specified time and perform the exercises carefully.

1. Arms Up on the Side: raise your hands making a 180° movement (2 minutes)
2. Shoulders rolls (40 seconds)
3. Biceps: arms parallel to the floor, come up at 90° angle (20 seconds)
4. Triceps on the chair: hands on the chair, push up to reach arms straight (8 repetitions) + shaking arms at the end (10 seconds)
5. Shoulders to the ears (45 seconds)
6. Hands Releases and Shakes (1 minute)
7. Neck left-right (1 minute) (Pg. 23)
8. Heels up and down (1 minute)
9. Leg up (hold for 5 seconds) and alternate with the other leg (45 seconds)
10. Hamstrings: sit straight, bring one foot behind and alternate with the other leg (50 seconds)
11. Hands on thighs and toes up (1 minute)
12. Goddess pose (Hold for 1 minute) (Pg. 39)
13. Shake legs and arms and breath in for 5 deep breaths (45 seconds)
14. March on the chair (40 seconds)
15. Step on the chair: go faster, alternating legs, (30 seconds) and slower (30 seconds) - 2 repetitions (2 minutes total)

Take a 1 minute break, drink a glass of water. Then repeat the very same sequence from Pose 1 to 15.

Final Stretching

Shoulders Rolls (15 seconds) (Pg. 24)
Stretching of the Chest (hold for 10 seconds) (Pg. 46)
Hands Stretching: open the hands and hold it there (1 minute)
Knee to Chest Stretching Left Side (30 seconds) - Right Side (30 seconds) (Pg. 34)

Breath and say Thank you!

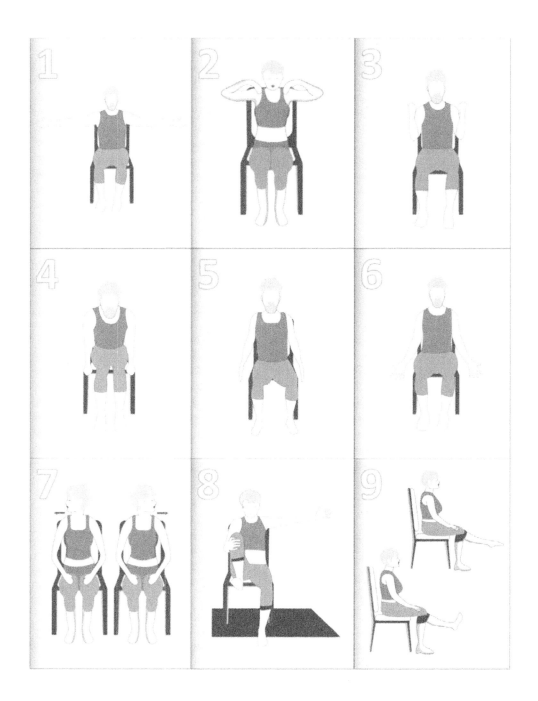

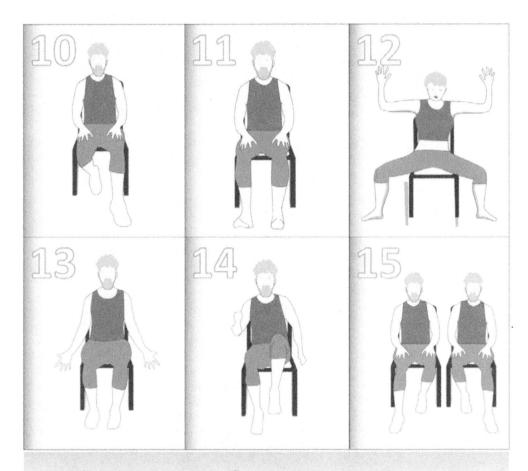

Repeat from 1 to 15

Final Stretching

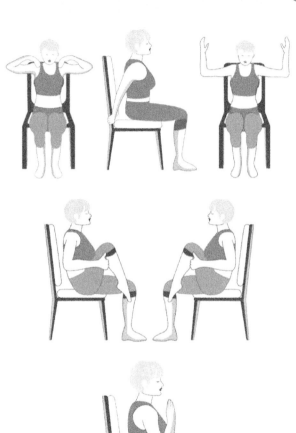

BOOK 7:
W4W:
WORKOUTS FOR WELL-BEING

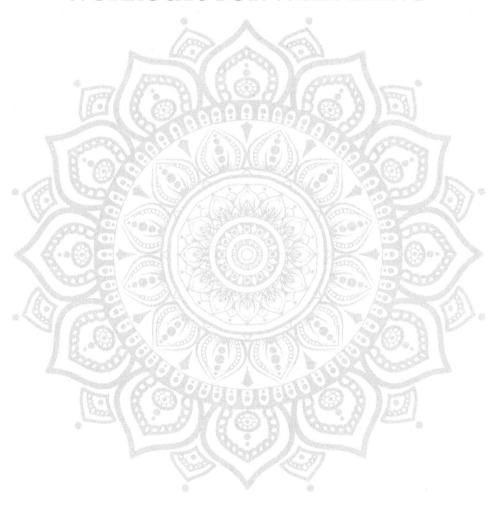

Chapter 1
Eternal Joy

By now, one thing is crystal clear: if we lead a sedentary life when we are elderly, we can face serious problems, also due to the weakening of bones and muscles, such as osteoporosis, fractures, for example, in the femur or pelvis, and develop circulatory disorders, including atherosclerosis.

This is why, for a person over 65, regular physical activity is essential, in fact:

• allows the muscles to remain elastic;
• activates and improves circulation;
• preserves the joints and strengthens the joints;
• promotes proper functioning of internal organs;
• it helps to counteract both physical and psychological chronic diseases, also reducing the risk of depression;
• contributes to mood, as it is an opportunity for socialization and interaction, and allows you to stay active in the body and spirit.

And here's how you can use this latest book: Whenever you have discomfort in one of the following body parts, open the book to the corresponding routine and do it!

Always remember that before starting, always ask your doctor for advice on any decisions about your health and movement. Good work!

Note: For reasons of practicality, I have collected the positions of the various flows in such a way as to have, at a glance, a general idea of what you are going to do for each of them.

My advice is always to study the positions and then, once you have made them yours, venture through the chapters of Book 7.

Finally, for convenience, for each flow, I have included the reference to the pages of each position scattered in the other books. Good workout!

Chapter 2
General Pain and Recovery Workout

Until 20 years ago, doctors recommended rest in case of back pain, but research over the years has shown that prolonged inactivity can worsen the situation; on the contrary, mild physical activity can greatly help promote healing.

Ideally, the activity should be aimed at developing endurance, strength, and flexibility; therefore, it can be useful to choose and perform:
- walking,
- running,
- riding a bike,
- some forms of dance,
- swimming,
- yoga or pilates;
- water aerobics.

In any case, it is recommended, before starting an exercise program, to talk about it with the attending physician, especially in case of major trauma or previous problems.

Regarding the exercises that we will see below, in general, it is recommended to:
- avoid sudden movements and, instead, always proceed slowly and gradually.
- also, pay attention to breathing, which should be as deep and slow as possible.
- feel moderate tension, in no case pain.

Some discomfort may be normal, especially during the first few sessions, but should improve over time with practice.

BOTTOM TO HEELS STRETCH

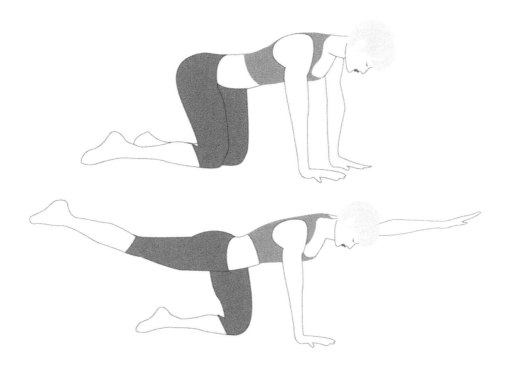

Kneel on all fours, with the knees level with the hips and hands under the shoulders.

Do not arch your lower back excessively. Keep your neck long, shoulders back, and don't lock your elbows.

Slowly bring your first leg backward, maintaining the natural curve of the spine. Hold the position for the time of a deep breath and return to the starting position.

Avoid pressuring your heels too much if you have knee problems.

Help yourself with a mirror to assume and maintain a correct position.

Don't force more than it feels. You can level up the exercise with the distension of the opposite arm.

Repeat 8-10 times.

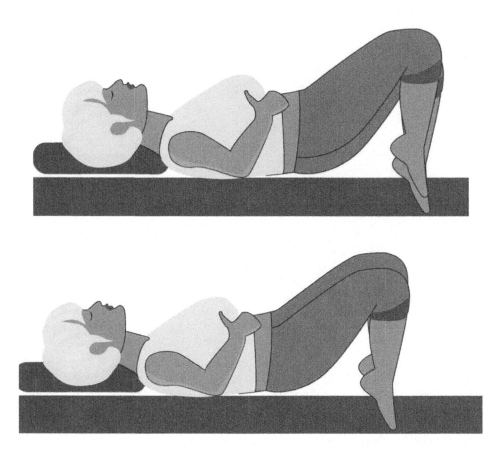

Place a small pillow under your head and lie on your back. Keep your knees bent and close together. Keep the upper body relaxed.

Rotate the knees to one side, then follow the pelvis, too, always keeping both shoulders on the floor. Hold the position for the time of a deep breath and return to the starting position.

Push only as far as you feel, without forcing.

Place a pillow between the knees if necessary to increase comfort.

Repeat 8-10 times, alternating sides.

BACK EXTENSION (COBRA POSE)

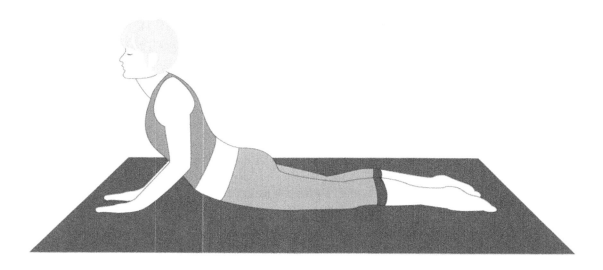

Lie on your stomach, leave your arms parallel to your body and bend your elbows, placing your palms at more or less level with your face.

Arch your back with force on your hands, keeping your neck straight. You should feel the tension in the abdominal muscles. Maintain the position for 5-10 seconds.

Do not bend the neck back.

Keep your hips on the ground.

The exercise can be done in many different ways, for example, by keeping the elbows supported or lifting them.

Repeat 8 to 10 times.

DEEP ABDOMINAL STRENGTHENING

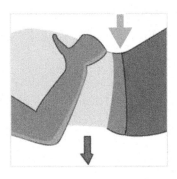 Lie on your back. Use a small pillow to rest under your head. Bend your knees and keep your feet straight. Keep your upper body relaxed.

During exhalation (i.e., while blowing the air out), contract the abdominal muscles (of the belly), creating an abdominal vacuum.

Hold this gentle contraction for 5-10 breaths, and then relax.

The exercise must be done gently, without forcing an excessive contraction.

Make sure you don't stiffen your neck, shoulders, or legs. In the second phase, you can also consider adopting a slight movement of the legs, as shown in the second part of the video. Repeat five times.

PELVIC TILT

Lie on your back with your knees bent, feet flat on the floor, and arms at your sides. Rest your head on a small pillow.

The feet should be approximately at the height of the hips, while the knees should be slightly closer to each other. Keep the upper body relaxed.

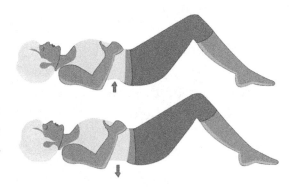

Gently flatten your back towards the floor and contract your stomach muscles. Then tilt the pelvis towards the heels until you feel the formation of an arch in the lower back accompanied by the sensation of contraction of the back muscles.

Do not apply pressure through the neck, shoulders, and feet.

Repeat 10-15 times, tilting your pelvis back and forth in a slow rocking motion.

Chapter 3
Water Aerobics General Workout

Like all physical activities, constancy is required for water gymnastics and at least two weekly training sessions. It is an excellent activity for your body, especially for those suffering from back pain or muscle aches, often generated by overweight and incorrect postures.

Furthermore, there are no age restrictions. Indeed, physical activity in the water is recommended for everyone, pregnant women, the elderly, people with disabilities, and people who need to undergo rehabilitation. It is perfect both for the exercises' simplicity and for the effort's adjustable intensity.

I know what you may think: finding the time to keep fit may seem impossible. Life can be so hectic, and we struggle to carve out the space to think about our physical well-being. Still, it's imperative that you succeed.

Try water gymnastics if gyms and traditional fitness activities can't break the stamina. The benefits are numerous, and it will take a few lessons to see the results on your body. Without forgetting that being in the water is a great way to relax, recharge your batteries, and face your daily tasks.

Do you still have doubts? The only way to find out if aerobic exercise in the waterworks is to try it. Dive into this experience; it could become your new healthy passion!

On the other hand, here are some specific workouts for the significant health problems and annoyances you may encounter over the years. I hope they make you feel as light and in connection with your body as I have experienced!

ARTHRITIS RELEASE WORKOUT FOR ANKLES, JOINTS, AND KNEES

WALK IN THE WATER

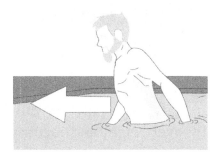

Stand in the waist or chest-high water, then walk 10 to 20 steps forward, then walk backward. Repeat.

For more resistance, increase the speed.

LUNGE FORWARD

Stand in the water at waist or chest height (near a pool wall for support, if necessary).

Take a lunge step forward without letting the forward knee pass your toes.

From the starting position, repeat with the other leg.

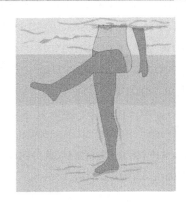

SIDESTEP

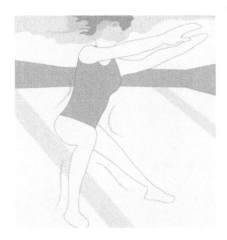

Stand in the water at waist or chest height, facing the pool wall.

Take side steps with both your body and your toes facing the wall.

Take 10 to 20 steps in the same direction and then return.

Repeat in the other direction.

HIP KICKERS

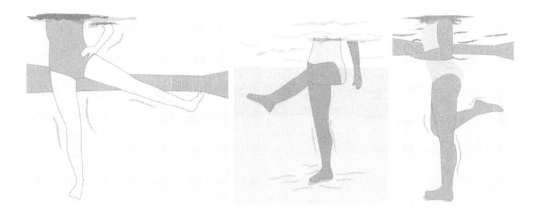

Stand in the water at waist or chest height, with the pool wall on the right side of the body as support.

Kick the left leg forward, keeping the knee straight, then return to the starting position.

Kick the left leg to the side, then return to the starting position.

Kick the left leg behind you, then return to the starting position.

Return so that the pool wall is on your right side and repeat the activity with the left leg.

JUMPING JACKS

In chest-high water, stand and bring your feet together and your hands by your side.

Jump astride your feet and bring your hands up to the water level, holding them in the water.

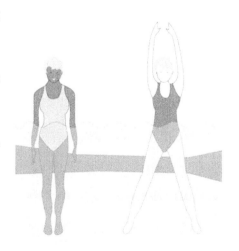

Return to the starting position, but repeat them as quickly as possible whenever you are ready.

For greater resistance, keep water foam dumbbells, slowing down the movements.

HACKY SACK

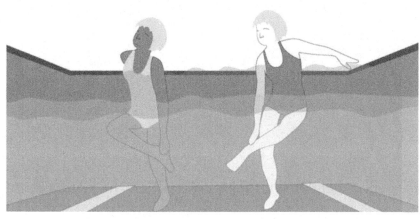

Stand in chest-high water.

Raise the right leg, with the knee bent, and the hip rotated open, and touch the inside of the ankle with the left hand.

Come down to the starting position, and repeat with the opposite side.

Switch sides as quickly as is comfortable.

FROG JUMPS

Stand in chest-high water.

Keeping the body in the water, quickly pull the knees towards the armpits (with the knees wide and the heels towards the groin) while

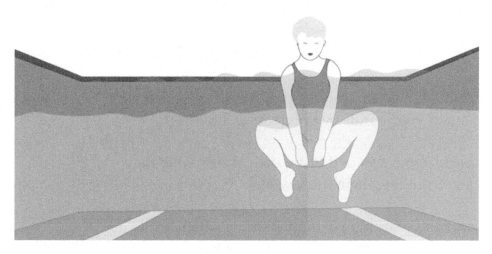

reaching the hands down to touch the feet as they rise to about the level of the hips.

Return to the starting position and repeat as quickly as possible.

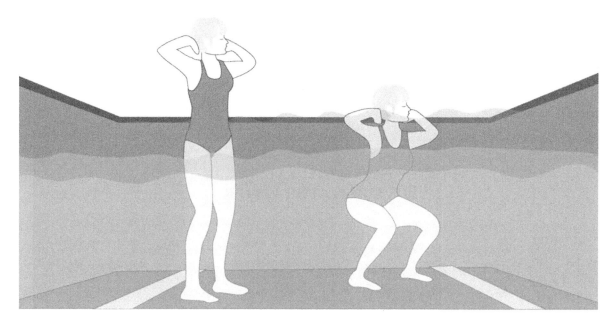

Stand in the waist or chest-high water.

Tilt your hips and bend your knees, lowering your body into a squat position with your arms forward.

Jump, coming out of the water, bringing your arms to the sides.

Stand on the balls of your feet and lower your heels, bending your knees and hips in a squat landing.

Repeat as fast as possible.

FROZEN SHOULDER WORKOUT

Exercising immersed in the pool can be of great help for the joints and, in particular, for the frozen shoulders.
Here are four simple exercises that I consider among the most effective in fighting pain by strengthening the shoulder muscles to make them more elastic.

ARMS UPWARDS

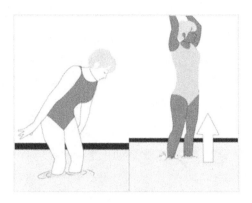

In the same position, start with the arms stretched at the sides, then bring them up, keeping the palms parallel or perpendicular to the ground, depending on the desired resistance.

The first few times, it is good that the exercises are not too hard.

DIVE INTO THE WATER

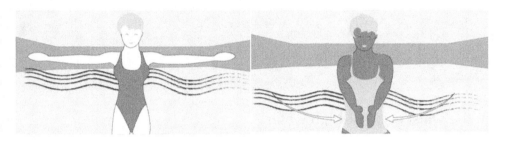

Start standing and with the water level with the shoulders, keeping the arms straight and the hands below the surface of the water.

Rotate the shoulders to bring the arms from parallel to perpendicular to the axis of the torso, then bring them back into the initial position.

FROM THIGHS TO HEIGHTS

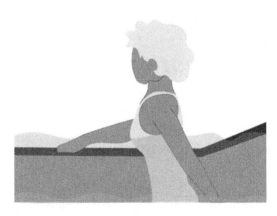

Standing as for the other exercises, keep your elbows close to your hips.

With your arms outstretched and palms on your thighs, bring your forearms up to form a right angle with your elbows.

It is also possible to modulate the water resistance by rotating the palm of the hands.

LOW BACK PAIN WORKOUT

WALK FROM ONE POINT OF THE POOL TO ANOTHER

Start at the end where the water is shallowest, no matter how low the level is.

Just enter the pool from the shallowest point and walk towards the deep water until you are submerged up to mid-chest.

Walking in the water is just walking back and forth in the pool, like in dry weather.

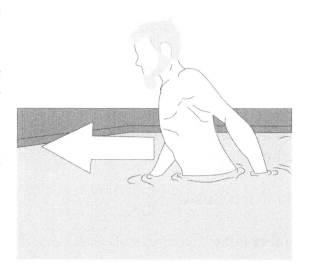

KNEE-TO-CHEST PUSHUPS

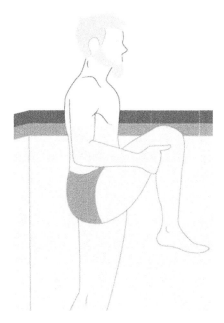

For this exercise, you must stay close to the pool's edge. Maintain balance by placing your right hand against the wall; the ideal is to stay immersed up to the chest.

Make sure that the right leg is the one closest to the wall. Shift your body weight onto this leg by bending the knee.

Lift your left leg by bending the knee, raising it as high as possible. Your goal is to bring the knee to the chest.

Repeat the movement 5 times for each leg.

'SUPERMAN' EXERCISE NEAR THE EDGE OF THE POOL

Stand in front of the wall with your hands resting on the edge.

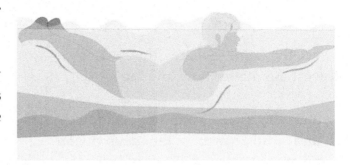

Slowly stretch the rest of your body backward while keeping your legs straight. You should assume Superman's stance while they fly.

For at least 5 seconds, hold the position before lowering your legs.

Do 5 to 10 repetitions.

Remember not to hyper-extend your back during the exercise.

PEDALING MOTION TO STRENGTHEN YOUR ABS

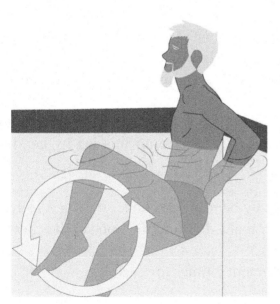

Rest your elbows on the pool's edge while turning your back to the pool wall. You need to stand in a spot where the water is deep enough so that you can move your feet without touching the bottom.

Bring your legs forward slightly and rotate them as if you were pedaling. In other words, raise one knee and rotate the foot forward, following a circular trajectory that brings it back.

The other foot should be simultaneously in the diametrically opposite point of the circle, turning forward and backward.

You can use this movement to move around in the water. Also, use your arms and let your feet move into the water. You can use a foam tube to support buoyancy.

UNDERWATER SQUATS

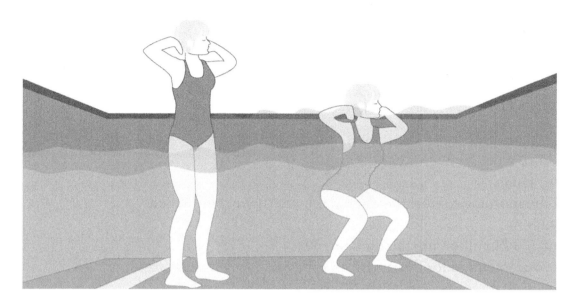

Spread your legs hip-width apart. Squat in the water by bending your knees and pushing your glutes back. You should reach a position similar to sitting. Make sure your knees don't go beyond the line of your toes.

Inhale as you squat; exhale as you stand up.

When you return to a standing position, ensure your abs are tight and your back straight.

During the exercise, bend the arms close to the body and the palms of the hands facing down.

Chapter 4
Back Pain Workout

Who: for you, when you have back pain.

What: your chair.

When: in the morning to start the day; in the afternoon; before bed.

Where: at home.

How: gently, without forcing the movements.

Why: set your intention for the practice: 'Today I choose this because ...'

Read the following instructions before starting.

Hold each pose for 5 deep breaths.

1.   Mountain Pose (Pg. 30)
2.   Cat & Cow Sequence (Pg. 31)
3.   Utkatasana (Chair Hands On Knees) (Pg. 39)
4.   Sitting Sun Salutation (Pg. 33; Pg. 35-36)
5.   Cobra Pose (Pg. 46)
6.   Twists - Right and Left Side (Pg. 51)
7.   Cobra Pose (2° repetition) (Pg. 46)
8.   Savasana (Pg. 43-45)

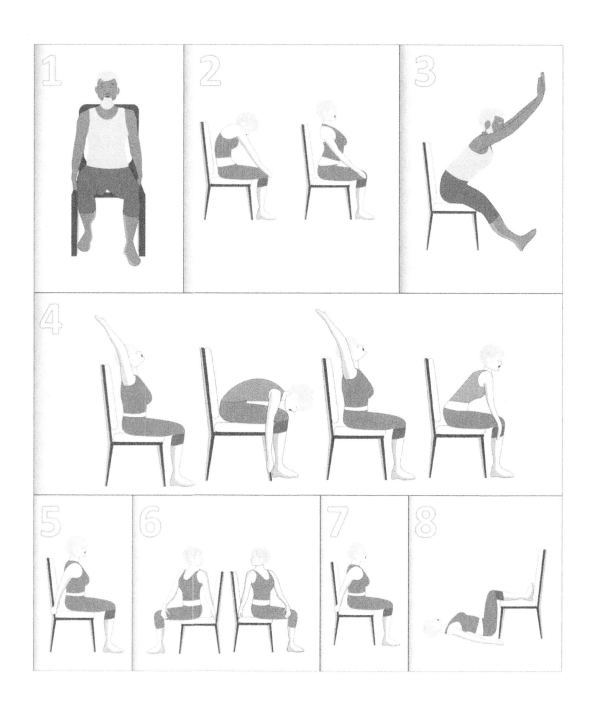

Chapter 5
Weight Loss Workout

Who: for you, if you want to promote your weight loss.
What: your chair.
When: in the morning to start the day; in the afternoon.
Where: at home.
How: gently, without forcing the movements.
Why: set your intention for the practice: 'Today I choose this because ...'

Read the following instructions before starting.

Hold each pose for 5 deep breaths.

1. Mountain pose (Pg. 30)
2. Anjali Mudra (Pg. 32)
3. Shoulders at the Ears (Pg. 24)
4. Neck Releases (Pg. 23)
5. Cobra on the Chair: Chest Out/Belly In (Pg. 46)
6. Cat & Cow (Pg. 31)
7. Raised Hands (Pg. 33)
8. High Altar - Right Side (Pg. 50)
9. High Altar - Left Side (Pg. 50)
10.Goddess Pose (Pg. 39)
11.Warrior I - Right Side (Pg. 52)
12.Raised Hands (Pg. 33) + Forward Fold (Pg. 35-36) (2 repetitions)
13.Pigeon Pose + Forward Fold - Right Side (Pg. 56; Pg. 35-36)
14. Goddess Pose (Pg. 39)
15.Warrior I - Left Side (Pg. 52)
16.Raised Hands (Pg. 33) + Forward Fold (Pg. 35-36) (2 repetitions)
17.Pigeon Pose + Forward Fold - Left Side (Pg. 56; Pg. 35-36)
18.Anjali Mudra + Ujjayi Breathing (Pg. 32; Pg. 21)

19. Hand on the Neck - Right Side
20. Hand on the Neck - Left Side
21. Palms on Belly - Final Breathing (Pg. 29)

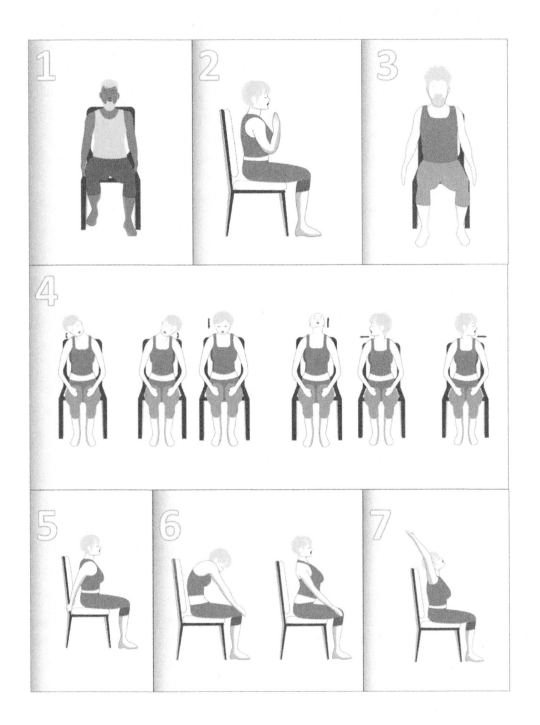

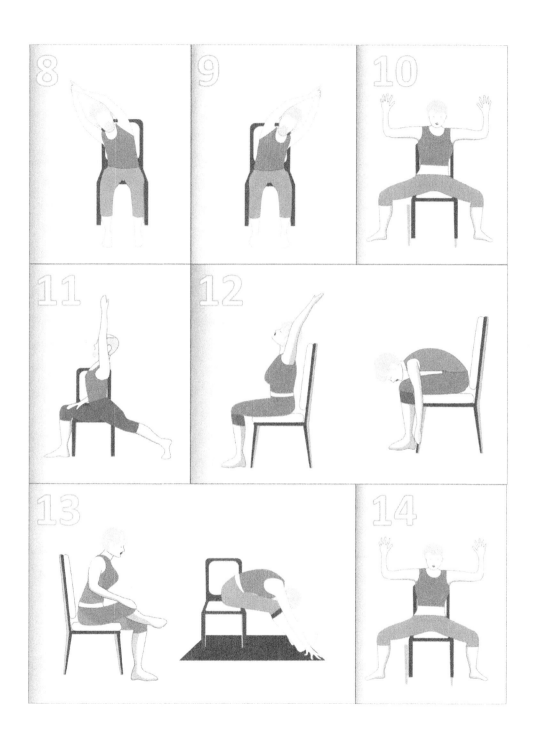

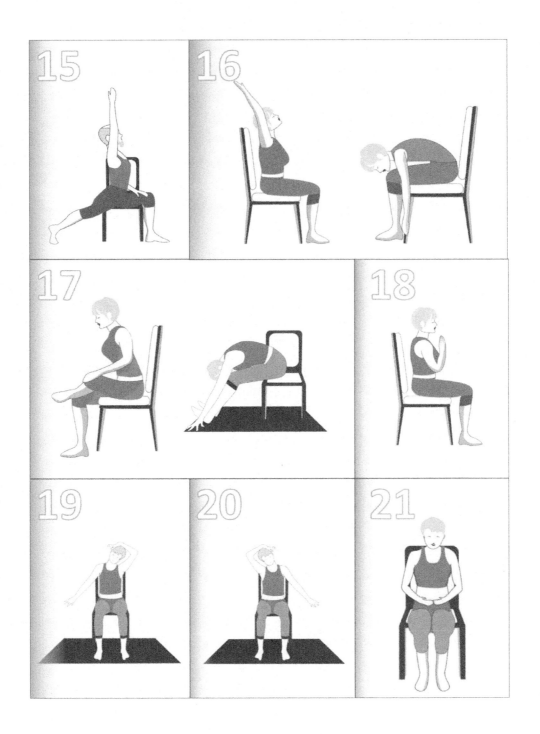

Chapter 6
Knee Injury Workout

Who: for you, when you suffered a knee injury and you are recovering.
What: your chair; a belt.
When: in the morning to start the day; in the afternoon; before bed.
Where: at home.
How: gently, without forcing the movements.
Why: set your intention for the practice: 'Today I choose this because ...'

Read the following instructions before starting.

Hold each pose for 5 deep breaths.

1. Hip Stabilization Exercise - Right and Left Side
2. Chair Flexing Foot Pose - Right Side
3. Chair Flexing Foot Pose - Left Side
4. Mountain Pose Chair One Leg Backlift - Right Side
5. Mountain Pose Chair One Leg Backlift - Left Side
6. Triangle Pose - Right Side
7. Triangle Pose - Left Side
8. On Knee Pose Strap - Right Side
9. On Knee Pose Strap - Left Side
10. Chair Flexing Foot Pose (2° repetition) - Right Side
11. Chair Flexing Foot Pose (2° repetition) - Left Side

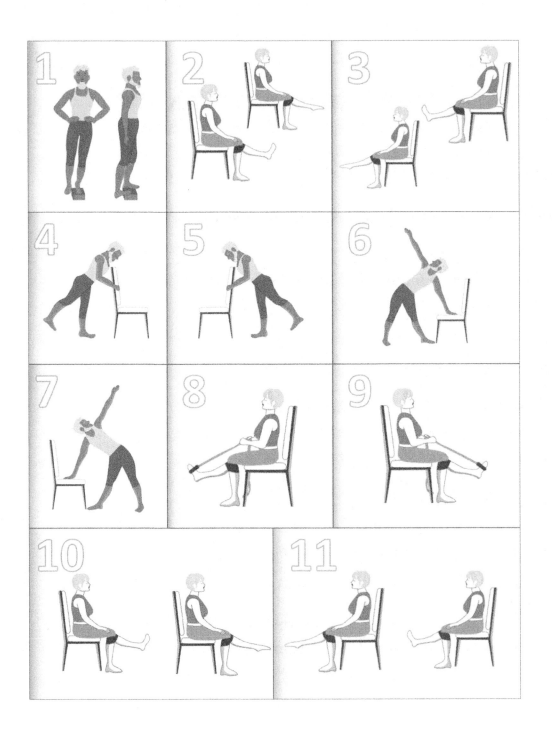

Chapter 7
Adaptive Yoga: Wheelchair Workout

Who: for you, if you are a wheelchair user.

What: your wheelchair; your bed. Just as Chair Yoga Poses, you can perform this flow both in your wheelchair and bed.

When: in the morning to start the day; in the afternoon.

Where: at home.

How: gently, without forcing the movements.

Why: set your intention for the practice: 'Today I choose this because …'

First thing first: come to a seated position in your chair, making sure that you're comfortable. You need to feel stable: do not forget to lock your brakes before starting the flow.

Also, make sure that your feet feel stable on our footplate: even if you can't feel them, they can give you excellent stability. When I try this flow with my students, we like to just wiggle around, ensuring our feet are providing us with stability.

Moreover, as we're sliding into our chairs a lot, we like to double-check that the but and the legs are just in the right place. Move around, adjust and find the stability to feel planted.

Then, start just focusing on your breath: close your eyes. As you take a deep breath, inhale, hiking the shoulders up to your ears. And as you exhale, you're lowering them down, pulling the shoulder blades together as they melt down your spine.

Follow the flow, and remember to hold each pose for 5 deep breaths.

Read the following instructions before starting.

Hold each pose for 5 deep breaths.

1. Mountain Pose on Wheelchair (Pg. 30)
2. Palms on Heart and Belly: Breathing on Wheelchair (Pg. 29)
3. Shoulders Rolls on Wheelchair (Pg. 24)
4. Side Bends on Wheelchair - Right Side (Pg. 37)
5. Side Bends on Wheelchair - Left Side (Pg. 37)
6. Twists on Wheelchair- Right + Left Side (Pg. 51)

Sun Salutation on Wheelchair (3 repetitions)
7. Raised Hands Up (Pg. 33)
8. Folder Down + Ragdoll on Wheelchair (Pg. 35-36)
9. Chair Chaturanga: press with your arms outstretched on the wheelchair, keep your back straight and compress your abdomen.

Repeat Poses n.7 -8-9 for (3 repetitions)

10. Right Hand Up: keep the hips down on the chair with opposite hand - Right Side
11. Left Hand Up: keep the hips down on the chair with opposite hand - Left Side
12. Raised Hands Up (Pg. 33)
13. Warrior 2 - Right Side (Pg. 53)
14. Raised Hands Up (Pg. 33)
15. Warrior 2 - Left Side (Pg. 53)
16. Mountain Pose on Wheelchair (Pg. 30)

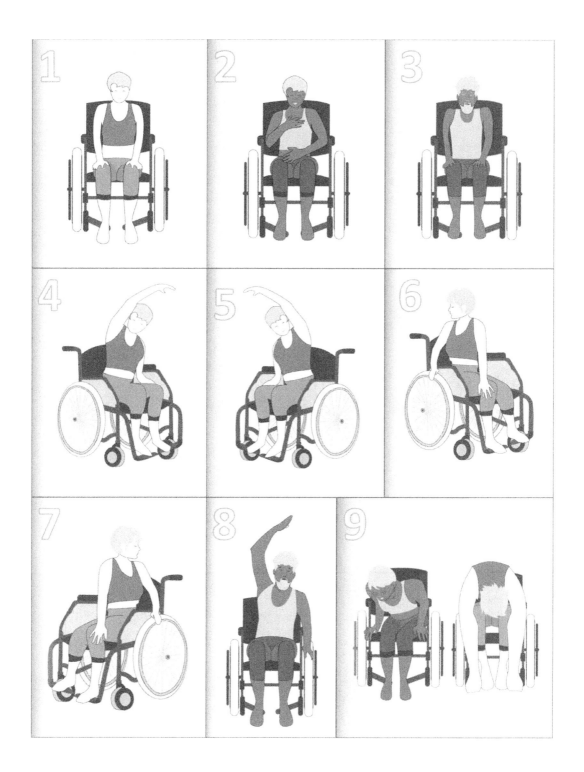

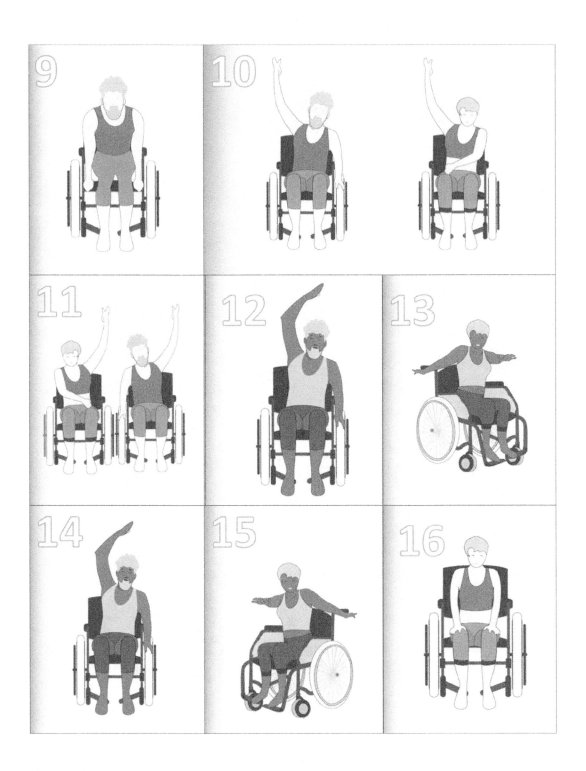

Chapter 8
Yoga for Arthritis Workout

Who: for you, if you have arthritis or osteoarthritis problems.
What: your chair.
When: in the morning to start the day; in the afternoon.
Where: at home.
How: gently, without forcing the movements.
Why: set your intention for the practice: 'Today I choose this because ...'

Read the following instructions before starting.

Hold each pose for 5 deep breaths.

1. Toes up and down
2. Ankles ups and down
3. Lift one leg - Right and Left Side (Pg. 27)
4. March in the place
5. Hips Circles
6. Stretch hips and flexors (Warrior I) - Right Side (Pg. 52)
7. Stretch hips and flexors (Warrior I) - Left Side (Pg. 52)
8. Seated Cat & Cow (Pg. 31)
9. Shoulders Rolls (Pg. 24)
10. Neck Releases: rolling in and out, chin to chest (Pg. 23)
11. Hands Releases (Pg. 124)
12. Raised Hands and Breathing (Pg. 33)
13. Side Bend Stretch Right Side (Pg. 37)
14. Side Bend Stretch Left Side (Pg. 37)
15. Cactus Pose (Pg. 37)

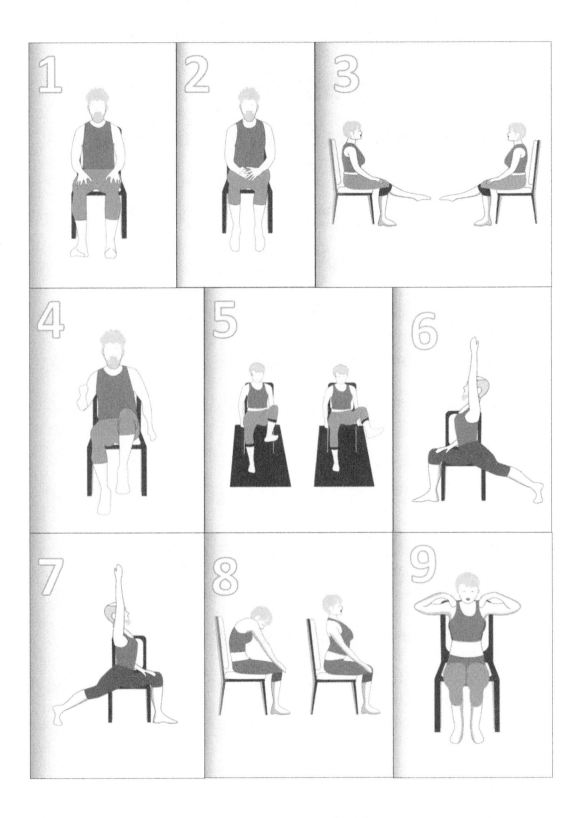

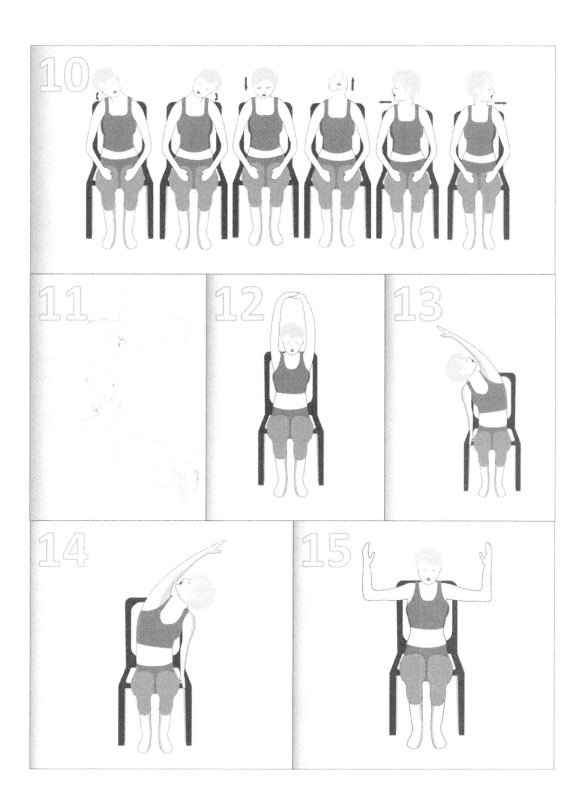

Conclusion:
Your Body-Mind-Spirit Journey

Here we are: we have come to the end of our journey together! Still, I'm not sad at all. And do you know why? Because your journey of building your renewed relationship with the body, the conscious and compassionate adventure within your mind, and witnessing the crystalline and 'light' balance of your soul has just begun!

In these pages, we have made many discoveries together. First of all, the fundamental importance of light but constant training as the first source of well-being in our senior years.

To guarantee a peaceful old age, we must think of our body and mind as a scale to be always kept in balance. It is not enough to train either just the body or just the mind. The ancient Latin expression *'mens sana in corpore sano'* has been widely misunderstood. The Romans knew that mental health had to be maintained as much as the health of one's body. We can say it: a holistic vision that surprises even today.

It is also necessary (sometimes I dare say 'mandatory') to pay attention to mental health, the balance of emotions, and the well-being of the body. For this reason, I believe that even in the life of the elderly, it is necessary to devote equal time to gymnastics of the body and exercises of the mind. Only in this way is it possible to improve one's general health and remain long-lived. On the other hand, staying young and fit for a long time is everyone's hope. Especially when you've had a stressful and busy working life and want to invest your retirement years as best you can.

So here, to conclude our journey in the best possible and helpful way, let's see how to organize your days and weeks with a mix of physical and mental activities to be included in the daily routine.

My Training Mantras

Training your mind for even just a few minutes daily can significantly impact you. I have collected some focal points that can help you train your mind and body by easily integrating them into your daily routine, apart from the habit of keeping this book on the bedside table or in the room where you train in order not to 'forget' your commitment and your compromise with yourself to love you and treat you accordingly.

• Train your body and stay active every day, even for a few minutes, especially in old age.

• More exercise means better mental health.

• Exercising your body becomes not a 'duty' but an inner need.

• More mental exercise means greater physical well-being.

• Train with a mix of exercises that keep your mind active and alert.

• Use every single book that you have found on these pages, learn calmly but consistently to perform each exercise you have encountered, and, finally, choose every day the flow, the muscle group, or the type of routine that 'resonates' with the mood or the demands of your body for that particular day.

• Your body intuition also works in choosing the ideal workout for you. Do not 'overdo' because your mind says so!

• Organize your week in the name of mind-body-spirit balance.

• Train your body and stay involved in old age wisdom.

My Weekly Choices

For physical exercise to have a positive effect (both on the body and the mind), it is scientifically demonstrated that it is always better to perform physical activity several times a week for not very long. 3-4 days are sufficient for a time not exceeding 45 minutes. Research has shown that more intense and prolonged physical activity can even adversely affect the body.
It would already be enough to dedicate a couple of hours of activity and physical exercise two days a week. Here are some examples for seniors:

• Gentle gymnastics;
• Tai-chi;
• Yoga;

- Slow walking;
- Group dances;
- Hiking;
- Sports in the water;
- Nordic walking;

All these different sports activities can also be distributed throughout the week. An example would be gentle exercise, slow walking, swimming pool sports, or hiking.

Three weekly activities are more than enough to maintain excellent health.

When you have pain in the hips or back, it is possible to alternate sporting activity with corrective physical action such as postural gymnastics. Many gyms are already fully equipped to receive the elderly for postural correction courses.

So, there are so many wonderful ways in which you can choose to take care of your wellness: here, you got to learn many valuable disciplines in your senior years, and also how to set up training routines, more or less intense workouts, and, finally, how to harmonize everything within a life full of love and serenity. And, of course, of inner and outer balance!

Welcome wisdom!
Namasté, Claudine

A Gift Before You Go...

If you missed it, Claudine thought of giving you a gift to amplify the experience of the book: a training journal to follow your workouts with awareness and fun!

Download it here using the QR code (in the image below) ...
and stay in touch with Claudine!

Made in the USA
Las Vegas, NV
11 March 2023

68925716R00195